This new edition of Juliette' … accuracy and clarity; new illu… making it substantially diffe… me name published by Faber … in1959.

Join **Juliette de Baira** … Gypsy, herbal veterinarian, and mother of two t… rs – as she spends an eventful summer swimming in the waters, and the history, of the Sea of Galilee, in the modern state of Israel. Juliette trains her observant eyes, and lovely descriptive prose, on the people, places, plants and animals around her.

You'll thrill as she and her children discover ancient treasures, be fascinated as she visits the tombs of Jewish mystics, hold your breath as Juliette dares to traverse the forbidden militarized zone around the Jordan River in pursuit of a personal communion with this holiest of lands, and, perhaps, scream in terror as she is visited in the dark of night by an enormous snake – only to breathe a sigh of relief when she is saved by her faithful Afghan hound.

Juliette vividly describes her visit to a Bedouin village, and the trouble this causes, both in the kibbutz where she lives and among the Bedouins. But with keen wit, steely nerve, and kind heart, she manages to please everyone, including her readers, as she saves the day and mends frayed tempers.

Praise for *Summer in Galilee*

"Juliette's personal bravery and respect for healthy simple living resonate strongly with me."
Ryan Drum

"Juliette is a wise woman and a great storyteller."
Isla Burgess

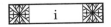

By **Juliette de Bairacli Levy**
from
Ash Tree Publishing
www.ashtreepublishing.com

Common Herbs for Natural Health
A Gypsy in New York
Nature's Children
Spanish Mountain Life
Summer in Galilee
Traveler's Joy

Summer
in
Galilee

Juliette de Bairacli Levy

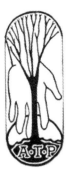

Ash Tree Publishing
Woodstock, NY

Ash Tree Publishing
PO Box 64
Woodstock, NY 12498
845-246-8081

www.wisewomanbookshop.com (to buy our books)
www.ashtreepublishing.com (to learn more about our
    books and authors)
www.susunweed.com (for more information on herbs)

Publisher's Cataloging in Publication
(Prepared by Quality Books Inc.)

Bairacli-Levy, Juliette de.
    Summer in Galilee / Juliette de Bairacli-Levy.
    Rev. and updated ed.
    p. cm.
    Includes index.
    LCCN 2005934397
    ISBN-13: 978-1-888123-06-7
    ISBN-10: 1-888123-06-0

    1. Bairacli-Levy, Juliette de. 2. Herbalists—Biography.
    3. Materia medica, Vegetable. 4. Medicinal plants.
    5. Galilee (Israel)—Social life and customs.
    6. Galilee (Israel)—Description and travel.
    I. Title.

RS164.B2922 2006   615'.321'092
                                        QBI06-600262

Table of Contents

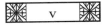

List of Photographs

All photos by Juliette de Bairacli Levy.

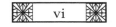

Introduction

Thirty-five years ago I was captivated by Juliette when I read on the dust jacket of her book: *"She is a busy farmer, botanist, practising herbalist, soil doctor, tree physician, wanderer in search of the sun, herb collector and anthologist of Gypsy lore."*

I was thrilled that one person could be all these things. But it was the wanderer in search of the sun that really got me! An ardent traveler and sun-worshipper myself, I treasured Juliette's words for their glimpses into her life with the Gypsies, peasants and nomads of different lands.

Under milk thistle, for example, she writes: *"The young shoots, called in Arabic* Khurfesh*, are gathered and eaten by the Bedouin shepherds and other Arabs. I have eaten quantities when living in or visiting Bedouin tents."*

I longed to know more about her times spent in Bedouin tents! But even then, thirty years ago, Juliette's travel books were out of print. I managed to find them in libraries and secondhand bookshops, and spent delighted hours in the reading of them.

Summer in Galilee is as lovely, enriching, and relevant today as it was 30 years ago when I first read it, and as it was 50 years ago when it was first published. It is lovely for its poetic writing, rich with little known details of the Holy Land, its plants and its people, and sadly, Juliette's passionate advocacy for peace and friendship between Jewish and Arab people is still relevant. Juliette, a Jewish herbalist who be-

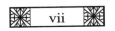

lieves in Christ, and who loves the Arabs, is the ideal person to show us around the Sea of Galilee.

It was *Summer in Galilee*, the first of Juliette's travel books that I read, that planted the seeds for my film *Juliette of the Herbs*. It was pure joy when I finally met Juliette and we began to wander in search of the sun – and good film locations – together.

As we roamed through Greece, Switzerland, France, Spain, and Portugal, we must have been quite a sight: two colorfully clad women walking through airports and villages with Juliette's typewriter, assorted bags carrying all her worldly possessions, my film camera and tripod, and Claire de Lune, the Afghan hound!

It was heavy work, but the magic of traveling with Juliette was everywhere. Owls flew by, Gypsies danced, fields of poppies waved, cows beckoned, nightingales sang. As we drove into Lanjaron, the village in the Sierra Nevadas where Juliette's daughter was born – now a large bustling town – we stopped to ask a woman directions to the old mill where Juliette had lived. She leaned through the window of our car and in sudden recognition exclaimed, *"Julietta!"* She was the sister of Rosario, the Gypsy who had suckled Luz as a baby! (See *Spanish Mountain Life*, Ash Tree Publishing.)

Of all the thousands of people in this busy town, we chose Rosario's sister to ask for directions. She took us immediately to Rosario's home, where Juliette was welcomed as the long lost friend she was; it had been forty years since Juliette and Rosario had last seen each other.

Read this book and away you go, traveling with Juliette and all the magic she brings with her: Hear the music of sheep, swim in Mary Magdalene's pool, taste sweet juicy pomegranates and freshly baked bread sprinkled with *Zahtar*, listen to stories of Maimonides, visit a Bedouin tent. Come, let's be on our way or, as Juliette says, *"Jal a drom."*

Trish Streeten, June 2010

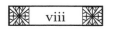

In Memoriam
Juliette de Bairacli Levy
11 November 1911–28 May 2009

Of all the remarkable women who have influenced me, the one I most identify with is Juliette de Bairacli Levy. She was a wild woman who ran with the wolves. She loved animals, especially dogs, goats, and bees. When asked to write an herbal for people, she famously replied: "They can use the remedies in my animal books" (*Herbal for the Dog*).

Juliette left veterinarian school and sought out the Gypsies of her native England (*As Gypsies Wander*). She learned well and applied what she learned with remarkable success. Her Natural Rearing Principles were proven with her prize-winning Afghan hounds, and by hundreds of vets.

Flaunting convention, Juliette had two children on her own (*Spanish Mountain Life*). She roamed with them and her hounds from country to country, settling for a season or two in places as diverse as the Sea of Galilee (*Summer in Galilee*) and Manhattan (*A Gypsy in New York*). In her later years, she lived on a small Greek Island, in Israel, in Germany, in many places across the USA, and in Switzerland (*Traveler's Joy*).

While I adore *Common Herbs for Natural Health*, *Nature's Children*, and *Herbal for Farm and Stable*, the book that lingers in my mind is Juliette's sole novel: *Look! The Wild Swans*.

Perhaps you are already a fan of Juliette's writing; perhaps you are new to her. In either event, I know you will be delighted, as millions of others are, with her wild wise woman herbalism and her ability to tell a tale. But be careful. You may become a wild woman, too.

Susun Weed, Laughing Rock Farm, 2010

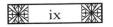

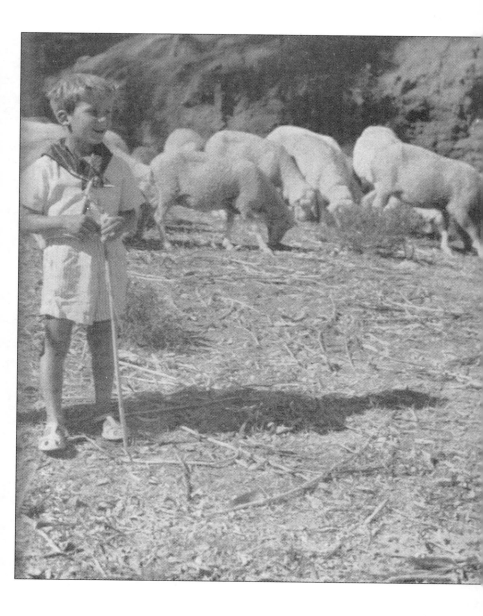

Rafik – shepherd

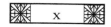

Chapter One

By the Lake of Galilee

Always I have tried to live close to water, by seas or lakes or rivers. This lifelong love for water brought me to Galilee in the summer time, to its lake, where there is water in abundance, close on thirteen miles in length and eight broad, with waters pure and limpid. It is said of lakes that they are imprisoned water; there is a sadness upon them, and a restlessness, and a yearning for the big rivers and the oceans. This I found true of the Lake of Galilee, only I found more; the special air of history over the lake itself, and all along its far-stretching shores.

Of this very lake in Galilee the ancient rabbis decided that God created seven seas, then he made the inland Sea of Genossar – Galilee – for his own delight, so that no other water on earth can be found to excel it in beauty and variety. After one summer in the hills of northern Galilee above the lake, and a further summer seven years later by that lake, I felt in agreement with the rabbis and also with the idea that lakes are waters held captive by the land.

The historical impression of the Lake of Galilee began with its signposts by the roads from the lake. They possessed such immortal names as Nazareth, Safed, Capernaum, Acre; and all around were the ancient camel routes leading to Syria, Lebanon, Egypt, and beyond. The camel roads were no longer used, except around Nazareth and Safed, and had become dusty wastes. But they could still be explored by my young boy and girl, Rafik and Luz, and I took them on numerous walks along those deserted places, peopled only with lizards as big as the common tortoise, and with the wayside dom trees which refreshed us with their small, berry-like fruits which taste like a mixture of dates and apples; these dom trees also give generous shade. Other travelers in ancient times must have enjoyed the dom trees, which are peculiar in bearing blossom and fruit at the same time on the same boughs, so that they seldom fail to offer food for all who pass by – man, animal, or bird. Like dates, dom fruits keep good for months, and therefore can be carried on far travels. The blossom is pungent with honey, and the whole tree is usually in song with bees and other insects.

Sometimes, as we explored, we found signs of the recent passing of camels, their great round footprints, sour-smelling dung, and often a scattering of dried tobacco leaves or corn from loads they had been carrying. We knew that the caravan roads led onwards from the Lands of Black Tents, the Bedouin people, east of the River Jordan which feeds the Lake of Galilee, to Egypt and Damascus. Now, along other newly made roads of concrete, went the heavy vehicles from the Israeli collective farms, or the army trucks and cars, only they did not go now to Egypt or Damascus while we were there, but kept to Israeli territory, owing to the prevailing hostility between most Arab countries and Israel; a pity indeed, with both races of the same Semitic origin and very close to each other in character, with their oriental blood.

A few times my children and I met with the camels themselves and their drivers. Those were all memorable meetings. The children would call out joyfully and run alongside the tall, tawny beasts, and wave their hands to the brown-faced riders who wore the flowing white *keffiyeh* with the black goat's hair *agal* braided around. And dark hands waved back and Arab faces smiled, for there is no man who does not enjoy welcoming greetings and admiration, even if it be Jew saluting Arab, as it was in this case.

The camels seemed to glide like the felucca boats of the swinging single sail as they went away over the sun-browned hills, their long necks weaving gracefully. Sometimes their saddles possessed trappings of brilliant colors, sometimes the camels wore big, clanging bells which echoed across the hills long after their wearers were out of sight. Once one of the cameleers threw down to us big pieces of sugar cane, several pieces for each. It was the first sugar cane that either Rafik or Luz had tasted. Like all children, they enjoyed that natural sweetmeat very much.

In former times there traveled those same caravan roads long files of mules carrying boxes and baskets of fresh fish from the Lake of Galilee for selling in Nazareth, Safed, and the more distant Acre and Jaffa, and taking also such fish, salted or pickled, to Jerusalem and even to Damascus. We never met with the fish caravans. I do not think that fish is taken in the former quantities from the lake. No one, while I was in Galilee, had seen boats sink beneath the weight of the catch in the nets, as happened in the times of the New Testament. Use of the lake waters for irrigation has diminished the fish population, as likewise have modern catching methods with the use of high-powered lamps to shine on the water and draw the shoals into nylon nets.

There are still a number of old water-side houses inhabited by Jewish fishermen and their families, and several places by the lake are in use as synagogues, but the greater part of the houses of Tiberias crowding close by the lake were wrecked, and their owners fled, during the War of Independence. There are few Arab families left in Tiberias now, and these who remain have mostly rendered good service to the Jews during their wars, and have thus been rewarded, or are Druze Arabs, who are a significant minority in Israel;

and with the establishment of the Jewish State were given the status of a separate religious community. The Druze are respected and liked by the Jewish people, for their hard-working and peaceful communities; and their agricultural villages remain in many parts of the mountainous regions of upper and western Galilee, prosperous and tranquil.

Those ruined houses by the lakeside are unpleasant places, stony heaps and piled rubble, and a sad air upon them found with most former homes destroyed in warfare. Few people go near them; they are the lairs of the half-wild dogs who became ownerless when the Arabs fled, outcast mating with outcast, and rearing their litters of lean whelps. Their food is the refuse of the city, and they eat by night, prowling in the gardens or yards of sleeping households. Those pariah dogs of Galilee are said to keep company with jackals, and when we eventually found accommodation in the old town of Tiberias, which is close by the lake, we had the old lake-side cemetery reaching to the back wall of our long and beautiful tree- and shrub-possessed garden, and we were warned not to enter the garden after dusk, as jackals had been seen there several times, their yellow eyes glaring in the darkness before they leapt back in to the cemetery where they prowled and thrust their pointed snouts into the graves, old or new, of Jew or Arab.

There can be few big cemeteries built closer to water than that of Tiberias by the Lake of Galilee. So close to the lake stands the cemetery that the sight of its crowding gravestones saddens bathers, unless they take the trouble and time to walk far enough away before going into the water. Over the area in springtime, crowd wild flowers, purple anemones and iris, as numerous as river reeds, and knee-high daffodils, pale-petaled as the big silver moths of the Galilean nights, but with trumpets the brilliant color of orange-peel.

By the Lake of Galilee

When I came to Tiberias with my children, I searched for accommodation by the lake, but at first found nothing. I was surprised by the poverty we met as we searched. Travelers in the past have written about the stinking alleys of Tiberias, with the crowding families, white-fleshed as ghosts despite the abundant sunlight of their land. Many of the places that we entered, *pensions* or private houses letting rooms, were like sordid scenes from French cinema: places of rattling keys and chains on broken-hinged doors, leading into unswept rooms dominated by rusted iron bedsteads with soiled mattresses.

Among the litter and dust upon the floor it was general to see the dead bodies of the big red cockchafers of which there are multitudes in Galilee despite all the chemical poison sprays used against them. The cockchafers lay on their backs in typical beetle manner, from which reverse position they had been unable to right themselves, and their bodies were peppered with the small black ants which are equally abundant in Galilee.

In the evil-smelling courtyards played naked, unwashed children, with running noses and matted hair. I refused all such accommodation offered, by saying that it was not modern enough, and stepped back thankfully into the clean, radiant sunlight. Therefore we went to live in the new town of Tiberias, known as Kiryat Samuel, built on one of the northern hills overlooking the lake, which itself is over 600 feet below sea-level. That proved a great mistake because the new town missed all the cool mists and breezes which arise from the lake, and likewise missed the fresh winds from the surrounding mountains which blow directly down onto the water but pass high over the new town. We also found the big cockchafers again.

We were accommodated in a clean, modern *pension*, for which we had to pay a big amount weekly for a small room, because, in Israel, tourists are charged for the number of beds occupied, not for the room itself, and my children and

I used three, it being impossible for the children to share a bed during the summer furnace heat of Tiberias, when most people who could afford to do so left the area until the weather cooled with the ending of the summer.

The ugly, scurrying cockchafers were everywhere; they even got into beds. Possessing wings, they could clamber up anything, house and room walls, and cupboards. I kept our room fairly free of such pests by pouring a strong-smelling mixture of herbs across our windowsill every night, and also across the door-tread. Such herbal odor did in some measure discourage the visits of the cockchafers.

The peculiar Tiberias cats catch and eat the cockchafers and other large insects. There seemed to be one or several cats to every Tiberias household. Small and thin, with very prick ears and whip-, rat-like tails, they live outdoors and are refuse-bin prowlers; mostly they run away at the approach of a human being, for they do not like human hands to touch them. Their sleek grace is admirable, and that is all.

There were two compensations for the lack of cool air in our Tiberias house and for the high cost of accommodation, and further the repulsive cockchafers: They were the view down to that lake of glorious beauty, and the abundant sunlight which entered our windows every morning from dawn until the mid-morning (by which time sunlight was not wanted) for bathing one's body in the golden light which feeds one's flesh and quickens one's nerves. In the later hours, when the heat of the sun has grown too fierce to give pleasure, it becomes an affliction.

Though the lake lay below, too far to give us the benefit of its cool breezes, still it was near enough for us to adore its beauty. Sometimes the waters were pearl-colored with heat, but very often they were possessed of all the blues, purples, and greens to be seen on the plumage of the kingfishers of Galilee, plumage which scintillated and shimmered in the light from the sun and reflected upwards from water waves.

I had only one month of sun worship in my *pension* room every morning, with my writing work accordingly progressing very well, when I was abruptly and completely deprived of that simple but valued pleasure!

There came to work at the *pension* a mattress cleaner. The *pension* was almost empty because of the hot season then upon Tiberias; therefore some seventy mattresses were available to the mattress man, and they were piled up almost directly beneath my window, where there was shade on the ground all the morning, from the balcony. The man's work was to fluff out the flock and remove the dust by beating all the flock from the mattresses against a harp-like instrument consisting of a steel cord stretched across a wooden bow, upon which a shuttle-like "hitter" was used. The fluff from the flock rose upwards in suffocating clouds, making it impossible to open windows even with the wire fly-protection-mesh across. The *pension* garden was filled with the flock debris and many of the goldfish in the pond were suffocated, despite my children's frequent cleansing of the pond surface, from pity for the fish.

That horrible mattress treatment began at six o'clock in the morning and continued for most of the day. Then a further disturbance was the opening up of numerous sacks of disgusting smelling chicken feathers wanted for filling pillows. The washing of the feathers created a repulsive smell which traveled far beyond the *pension*.

Our remedy was to leave the place at once, but it was not possible to do so because our money, long overdue, had not arrived. I had barely enough to feed my children, nothing at all for the expense of removal with much luggage. Late arrival of money, as I traveled, was a frequent event and seems to be experienced by most of my writer and artist friends who work outside their countries of birth. In the Tiberias *pension* I had not minded living for weeks on less than half the food supplies which I used at other times; I had not minded while I had the sun to feed me daily. Then, deprived of the sun, and with the flock dust choking our lungs, we really suffered. It became impossible to do any writing, for which some peace of mind is needed.

Therefore I took my children to the lake from early morning until dusk, by which time the mattress man had left the *pension*. He always went away looking like a snowman, his uncovered head, his ragged body, coated with white fluff. Although Rafik, Luz and I considered the man our enemy because he brought the dust with him, we pitied him his horrible profession. He was a Tiberias man, we were told, and in that pitiless heat he passed the days and years of his life, seated upon the ground, choking his lungs and pricking his skin with the dust and dirt clouds which he created.

We endured the mattress man and his work for nearly two weeks, and then one morning a swallow entered through an open skylight window of the *pension*. It was seeking exit, darting in its distress to and fro across the high ceiling for some while, until I found a helper with a ladder and had more windows opened to aid the bird's escape. I was convinced that the swallow's coming was a good omen for me: It has always been so when swallows have entered a house where I have been living, and where they have no nest or reason for entry. This again proved to be so, and within two days of having the swallow in the *pension* I received the delayed money, and we left the unpleasant place in which poverty had kept us over-long.

I was happy because, after much search, I had at last found a room close by the lake itself, close enough to enjoy the refreshing cool breezes off the water, and to feel that we were part of the lakeside life, the sounds and scents, and the rhythm of that great stretch of water – even if the cemetery now stood quiet and sad outside our garden.

Now we could watch the fishermen from the lake hanging out their nets to dry in our nearby grove of eucalyptus trees. Some fishermen used nets of nylon, pleasant enough to look at in their colors of buff or rose or gray. I preferred, though, the old-type ones of dark string, with their necklaces of pale corks. They made the more graceful shapes as they draped across the eucalyptus boughs, with the big blue kingfishers or the white and black ice birds flighting above them, and the sun dapples from the tree foliage reflected on their brown mesh, through which, veiled and mysterious, views of the lake could be seen, and also, across the waters, the feet of the hills beyond.

For added measure of enjoyment, that eucalyptus grove, amongst the coolth and the patterns from sun and foliage, and the graceful nets, was a meeting-place for swallows. One does not associate swallows with trees; their feet are not formed for resting on branches. Nevertheless, they thronged in the grove and were like many more leaves upon the graceful branches, and they quickened the air with their twittering, which was most sweet to hear.

The owners of the *pension* by the lake where we found our new living-place, were away during the hot season, and a family with many children took care of the big old house. Mme Avigdor, the mother, spoke good French in addition to the Hebrew and Arabic generally spoken in Tiberias. She had lived some time in Corsica and learned her French there. I came to like her very much.

She was an expert needle-woman, and as she sat long hours at her sewing machine, she would tell me legends concerning Tiberias, of which she knew many. She had an especially good store of legends associated with the lives of the many great rabbis who once lived in Tiberias during the great Roman-Jewish wars, and who are mostly buried there, and give much of its fame to that capital town of the Lake of Galilee.

Summer in Galilee

She made a dress as a gift for my daughter Luz, and it came in the color of an evening primrose, piped with royal blue.

Although our room balcony overlooked the main road south out from Tiberias, we slept there on that balcony; the nights were unbearably sultry by that time of the summer, and when the old stone of the house gave out its heat absorbed from the sun during the day, the interior then had the heat of an oven.

It is always a pleasure for me to sleep outdoors, and it is an especial pleasure in those warm, windless, star-possessed nights of Galilee. When I rented the balcony room it was early August, and the Galilean summer was at its meridian. But every night outdoors was cool, with the breezes from the lake rising to us and fragrant with the breath of the night-scented jasmine which trailed over the old walls near our balcony. That balcony faced the Great Bear constellation, and to look toward those stars from my bed has long proved to be another good omen for me. We found happiness in our new home, and every night, after days by the lake, my children and I lay on the cool balcony and watched the Mediterranean stars flashing in the grape-purple sky.

Below our room was a street lamp, and at all times of the night bats and huge moths could be seen spiraling around it, the moths kissing their love, the lamp, and then dying from its burning touch. Big tawny salamanders also could be watched as they moved swiftly up and down the wall against which lay our bed mattresses, which I placed nightly on the balcony floor. The salamanders watched us with their brilliant sequin-like eyes, and then dropped their mouse-like dirt pellets onto our coverlets!

One night there was music below our *pension*. A man sat on a milestone at the roadside below us, while he seemingly awaited transport to take him away along the South Road. As it was a Sabbath night very little traffic was on the roads. As the man sat waiting on the milestone he played country tunes on an Israeli flute of woods so dark that it looked like ebony. The man was young, not handsome, although well built and interesting looking. His real beauty were the slim, supple hands holding the flute, upon which the lamp shone down. The tunes of the player heard from my balcony were all sad, if sweet. I wondered who the player was, and from what country he had come – as one always wonders in modern Israel, with its teeming immigrants – and to where he was going.

Soon the man noticed me and the sleeping children, and then he was playing his tunes for me, and that was yet more enjoyable. His eyes met mine often; laughing eyes he had, though his music was doleful. I did not speak, he did not speak. Speech would have spoilt the music. I was happy to have the player there, and I hoped selfishly that transport would be long delayed in coming to take the player away.

Mme Avigdor, having heard the music, came to my room from her own, and to my balcony. When she saw that the music was for me, she smiled at me, waved her hand at the player and me, and went away.

Soon after, a big kibbutz lorry came along, going south. The driver saw the man waiting on the milestone in the late night and stopped; the player clambered in. The stranger waved his flute back at me from the lorry and I waved back and called out my thanks for his tunes. I did not expect that I would see him again: he and his music would be one memory from a hot, jasmine-scented, summer night in Galilee.

Of much interest to us were the sheep and goats pastured on a long lakeside strip of land facing our veranda, and across the road beneath us. There was shade from date palms and willows, and a fair amount of rough grazing. The flock was herded by an old shepherd who managed them all

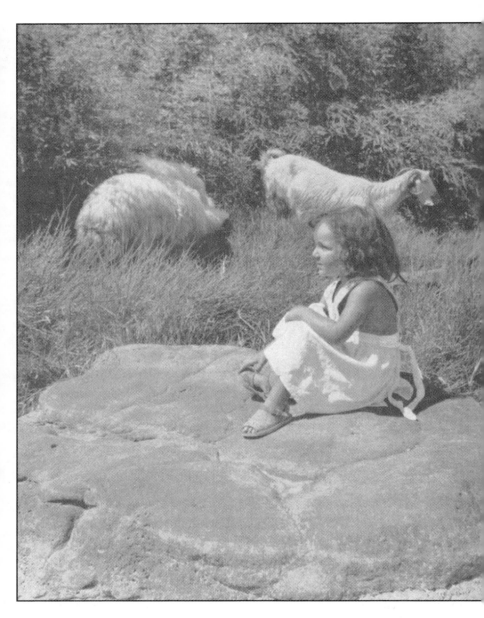

Luz and goats amongst the willows of Galilee

with skill. The shepherd resembled pictures of patriarchs of the Bible: tall, thin, and dark-skinned, with long strands of white hair pushing under his brimless hat, around which he sometimes wound a white cloth to look like a turban. His nose was Semitic and shaped like the crook he carried; his white beard was pointed and goat-like. His clothes also were white, and he had thin and curved black-skinned legs, resembling carob fruits beneath the knee-length, baggy trousers. On windy days he wore a dark cloak to protect his aged body from the dust storms, despite the heat. On days of very fierce sun a broken straw hat was added. For Sabbath days he appeared splendid in clean white garb. He kept the Sabbath strictly, and from Friday afternoon until the Sunday early morning he handed his crook to another shepherd, and did no work for the flock at all.

The Sabbath-day temporary shepherd was of very different type to the regular one, being big and fat and florid. His head appeared abnormally small because of the contrast with his huge stomach — which he carried well before him and which seemed to spread from the place where waist would be, right down to the knees. "Round like a watermelon in front," my children commented. They did not like the Sabbath worker, for their watchful eyes observed that he bullied the animals in his care. The flock in turn played truant with the fat man, running away to the lake, or trespassing on the main road.

A young bullock was added to the animal company and was kept tethered beneath a willow tree in the shade.

"Doesn't it want to walk about and use its legs in running like we do?" my children asked. The bullock seemed to love the old shepherd, for it lamented for hours, with loud bellowing, every time the man left him to take the flock farther away out of sight. The young bullock sensed or scented the shepherd well before he appeared, and the animal's excited bellows could be heard far off. "The shepherd is coming!"

Rafik and Luz would tell me in excitement. They worried also about the creature's loneliness. And glad the bullock was at the keeper's return, rushing playfully at the old man to the full length of the rope which held it, its big head tossing and its tail raised high.

From our veranda we became on calling-out terms with the old shepherd, and his coming and going with his beautiful animals was of daily interest. Yet we were puzzled because the animals were being changed almost weekly. Black and white goats were replaced by tawny, a pair of black-streaked ewes went, and a big white ram came in their place. Then the bullock which had become part of our daily life by the lake was missing, and we never saw it again. It did not seem a proper herd to us, with the animals changing frequently; we did not know enough Hebrew at that time to ask the shepherd for an explanation.

Then one Monday morning we were given the solution to the strange character of the flock. A flat-cart went by, beneath our veranda, laden with goats held down by ropes so that they lay on their sides. Live goats? No! Not all alive! Two white dead ones lay amongst the living, the necks of the white ones drooping like swans. On the end of the cart sat the fat man, whom we knew from the herd, his thick legs hanging over the side. That made it obvious to us. The fat man was a butcher, and the cart with the fair goats, dead ones cruelly put with the living, was going to the slaughterhouse, a white building which stood back from the lake a short distance on the south side. The old shepherd, therefore, who tended his flock with such loving care, was employed by the butcher, and all the animals which we watched daily from our window, including the beautiful black and white goats and the loving sentimental bullock, were merely being prepared for slaughter, fattened on the lake shore herbage almost within sight of the slaughterhouse awaiting them all with its terrible atmosphere of violent deaths, to afflict the sensitive nervous hearts of the herbivorous animals before their own moments for being slain came to them. It was a sad discovery! We therefore booed the butcher as he drove by beneath our balcony. He did not hear us, and would not have understood if he had heard. My children and I could protest rightfully against those animals going to their deaths, for, as vegetarians, we took no part in eating anything from slaughterhouses.

After a further time of watching more animals come and go, my children and I were hating the butcher. I tried to take no more interest in the herd, pretending to myself, and having my children pretend likewise, that there were no animals being pastured on that lake shoreland which faced us. But, as we loved very much all goats and sheep, such pretense proved difficult.

Then the butcher himself took charge of the herd for more than a week, the old shepherd not appearing at all. By the end of that time, Rafik's antagonism — encouraged by his young sister — towards the man who bought, fattened, and took to their deaths so many animals, seemed to have gotten beyond the child's control. An incident happened by the Lake of Galilee which I shall long remember.

We were without bread one day and I had to go to the town to purchase more. I left my children playing with hoops in the pleasant and shady garden of the *pension.* I passed by the butcher in his usual place on the land facing our veranda. He had no sheep with him, only many goats of many kinds, including a trio of the beautiful black-and-tan type with shaggy legs, which I had first seen and admired in the Bedouin village of Toobah on my previous visit to Galilee. There was also a young calf, milk-white, patched with bronze: very fair to watch as it gamboled with the goats. I tried as always to pretend to myself that I had not seen the animals: that they were not there, that I had only imagined them. But passing close to the animals I saw them too well, and I sorrowed.

On my way back from the shops, as I approached the *pension*, I was surprised to see that Rafik had departed from the security of the garden where I had left him, and had crossed the dangerous main road along which there was no speed limit for the thronging vehicles of all kinds, and there he was amongst the goats and sheep and, moreover, he was stoning the butcher! The little boy, flute in one hand and big stones in the other, was quite close to the big bulk of the butcher as he flung the stones at him. But the missiles coming from a small boy, in a seemingly very angry state, failed to reach their target. The astonished and enraged butcher was likewise flinging stones, only smaller ones.

At a window of the pension stood Mme Avigdor, shouting at the butcher not to harm a child who was a stranger in the land; she was also shouting at Rafik to return at once. I hurried to my boy and took his hot dusty hand and led him away, telling him that I was disappointed that he had broken his promise to me never to cross the dangerous main road alone.

Rafik's explanation was that he had had "a plan." Like the Pied Piper of Hamelin (a story known in every detail by my children for – having myself suffered from broken promises of others – we had much sympathy with the Piper of Hamelin), he had planned to pipe the goats and sheep away from the butcher and take them to safety in the hills far from the slaughterhouse. He had piped a long time on his flute but the herd had not followed. Only they had ceased their grazing, and watched the stranger among them. This interruption of the animals' feeding seemingly had annoyed the butcher, who wanted his charges to achieve the maximum fatness for slaughter; and he had shouted at Rafik to go away: words of Hebrew which the boy well understood. And the boy, desperate at the failure of his "plan" and also antagonized by the butcher's violent shouting, had begun throwing stones.

A nicer memory of shepherding by the Lake of Galilee was given by "The Little Shepherd Boy" – as my children called him. It was a pleasure to see the slight boy skillfully controlling the big, unruly herd of half-wild goats which included several big bucks. Thin and dark he was, and in his speech and manners possessed all the politeness of another world, an older, less cynical one.

And he shepherded a real herd, not merely a group of animals being fattened for the slaughter. Month after month we saw the same animals grazing along the north shore of the lake. Black and silver they came, tawny and brown, pied and streaked, smooth-coated or shaggy, and with ways as wild as goats from higher far mountains beyond Galilee. They sprang with the grace of great birds from rock to rock by the water, snatching at the green grass which pushed up between many of them where use of the lake for irrigation, also sun evaporation of the waters in the midsummer, caused the water line to recede a considerable distance from its natural place. The goats rustled the willows as they pulled at them, and sent the thronging butterflies soaring away like airborne blossoms from the wild buddleia, vetches, and a sweet-scented species of hawthorn. In the same way as ourselves, the goats liked to be on the lake rocks in the early morning sunlight. They seemed to be in a state of dream, with their gray-green or topaz eyes half-closed, their finely horned heads nodding as they knelt there.

The shepherd boy went by over the rocks, as fleet-footed as his goats. He wore an old brown leather jerkin and tall boots, despite the heat, and had the look of a young goat himself; his eyes, too, were long and slanting, slits of light flashing in his sun-blackened face beneath a thicket of curling black hair. His name was Haim; he was a Jewish shepherd, Palestinian born, and spoke Hebrew and Arabic.

Rafik and Luz loved the boy, and soon began keeping things for him; grapes and plums, and a portion from their small rations of sweets and sugar biscuits, especially that delicious oriental sweetmeat, halvah made from sesame oil and honey. All the time that we knew Haim, the high cost of food in Israel made our own supplies very short, but as my children derived much pleasure from putting aside portions for "The Little Shepherd Boy," I let them do as they wished.

It was difficult to get Haim to accept things. He obviously enjoyed the gifts, but it was part of the almost daily "Little Shepherd Boy" game to go through a half-hour or more ritual of laughing refusal before acceptance was finally granted, and the fruit and sweets eaten. Rafik and Luz enjoyed every minute of that game, which always had the same happy ending. Sometimes "The Little Shepherd Boy" kissed Luz; then her face turned the pink of damson blossom from her pleasure and pride.

Haim was charming with my children. He would catch hold of the shaggy manes of his half-wild goats and lead them up to Rafik and Luz for them to caress them and feed them crusts of bread or handfuls of grass; and he never failed to bring our favorite, a white, black-headed female kid. One morning Haim came calling to us joyfully down the hillside, carrying in his arms a new kid, a baby of fawn and white color, with eyes long and dark, much like those of the shepherd boy himself. Haim told us that the kid's mother had died and he was rearing it by hand, and it could now eat non-milky foods very well. What was touching was the way that the baby goat called and cried after the boy, as a kid after the nanny. Whenever Haim went out of range of the kid's eyes it would be crying out to him and he would be replying to the very voice of a goat.

'N-eer-eer-eer,' one would call to the other, one frantic, the other comforting, there by the beautiful shining waters of the lake − all of us keeping company there with kingfishers, ice birds, dragonflies, and species of orange and white butterflies, big and small ones, called in Galilee

"The Ladies of the Lake," the "Great Ladies of the Lake," and the "Little Ladies."

Those foothills around the Lake are still sheep land. There on our wanderings we met many shepherds with their flocks, and especially notable were the black-faced sheep of the golden, intelligent eyes.

The shepherds were often aged men of typical Old Testament type, with thin sun-charcoaled faces, arms and legs, and wearing flowing white robes, with a scarf headdress of Arabian style.

The sheep bells by the lake were pleasant, tolling music, distant or near. When near, they had the accompaniment of the zither sounds of the grasshoppers and the siffling of the sun-brittle grasses and reeds as the lake airs stirred them, coming and going in their mysterious infrequency.

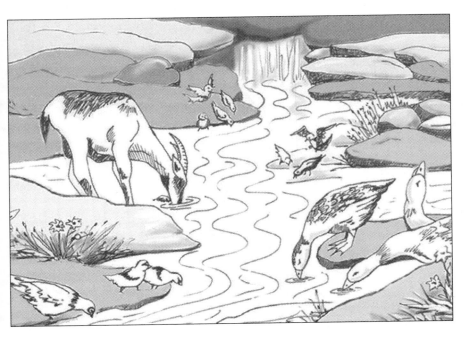

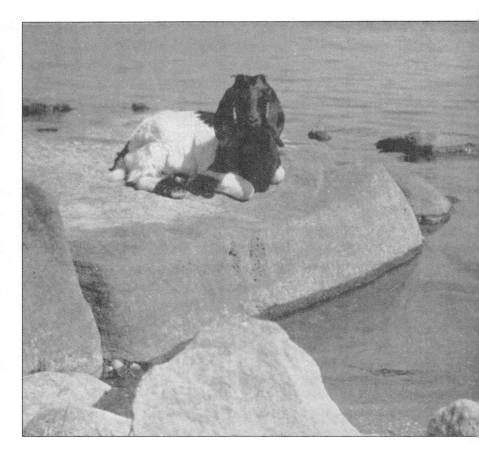

The black and white goatling

Chapter Two

The Lake of Galilee

For beautiful things men have many names, and that inland Sea of Galilee possesses names as many as pearls on a fine necklace.

The neighbor lake to the Sea of Galilee – the Dead Sea – is joined by the same River Jordan, but, so far as I could find, has only one other name, the Arabic one of *Bahr Lut.*

But the Galilee! the shining limpid waters where the music of the waves mingles with the voices of birds, and around which towering hills as beautiful as the lake make a circle, is a sea made not only for God's own delight (as the rabbis said), but also for the delight of humankind from the beginning of the world to the present day. And humans have praised it with many names.

The lake's geographical name is the Sea of Galilee; then further there is the geographical Israeli name of *Kinnereth* – the Harp – derived from the harp-like shape of the great stretch of water as seen when looking down upon it from the hills. The Arabs call the lake, *Bahr Tubariya,* after Tiberias. Old maps name it as Lake of Genesaret, also Genezareth, Lake Galilaeal, Sea of Genossar, Sea of Chinnereth, Sea of Tiberiadis, and Sea of Taricheal.

And poets have other names for this lake: The Handmaiden of the Mountains, The Jewel, The Silver

Woman, The Blue Harp, and simply: The Sacred Lake. The oldest and most famous name seems to be that of Galilee, from the Graecized form of the Hebrew *galil,* a word found in the New Testament in I Kings, 6:34, meaning "the folding or rolling of a door," or "circle," and translated as "a ring" in Canticles 5:14 and in the Old Testament, in Esther 1:6. And it is well descriptive, for hills encircle the lake.

The people of Tiberias always call it "the Sea," and speak of "going to the Sea." Except during times of storms – with the waters of the Harp lashed up into high waves and with an ocean's fury and power – that thirteen-mile stretch of water was always a lake to me: its bird, fish, insects, and shore-side flowers are all things of a lake, and in my writing that is what I call it.

All who speak or write of this glorious water of Galilee make the place female, and those who know the lake well, living by it or fishing on it, declare that only a feminine thing could be so changeable: that water calm, and smooth as new cloth one hour, then wave-possessed and seething the next. These squalls occur with rapidity, and because they are dangerous to the fishermen caught out on the lake, send all the boats racing to the safety of the shore-side.

The fishermen say of the lake that her tides and currents, and the fish within those waters, are all much influenced by the moon, and that only female things are so wooed by the moon and so moon-possessed. Those sudden and violent-tempered storms which blow through the gullies between the encircling hills are dreaded by the lake fishermen, as likewise they were in the time of Peter and his brother fishers.

Nowhere are there better descriptions of the Lake of Galilee storms than in the New Testament; the calm that comes after the quick tempests, for instance:

> And there arose a great storm of wind and the
> waves beat into the ship, so that it was now full.
> And he was in the hinder part of the ship asleep

> on a pillow; and they awake him and say unto him,
> Master, carest thou not that we perish?
> And he arose, and rebuked the wind, and said un-
> to the sea, 'Peace; be still.' And the wind ceased and
> there was a great calm. (Matt. 8:24–26)

My children and I witnessed many such storms over the Lake of Galilee, with the waves rising to heights which flung them halfway up the trunks of the shore-side eucalyptus trees — most of those trunks taller than thirty feet — and the silver spray of the flinging waves reaching the delicate down-hanging foliage.

The lightning, which was a frequent presence in the lake tempests, came closer to my children and me than we had ever met with elsewhere, some flashes so close that we flung ourselves back from the lake in fear: for we liked to bathe in those storms with the cool rain — a joy in that torrid climate — streaming down over our heads and bodies. Those times made the lake appear true to its other name of "the Sea." And people who know the lake well have told me that storms on the Lake of Galilee are as dangerous as on any sea, possibly more dangerous, because the waves have a whirl and a suck in them which overturns boats and drowns bathers.

In connection with the violent squalls, Mme Avigdor told me about the old fishing days on the lake, of the times when the waters teemed with frail Arab fishing boats. When the Galilee storms lifted and flung those boats about, the Arabs would pray for their salvation — not to Mohammed their prophet, but to the great Jewish Rabbi: Rabbi Meir Ba'al Ha-Nes, whose name, meaning Miracle-maker, was bestowed on him by his disciples, and whose tomb, housed in a lofty memorial building on the southern shore of the lake (close by the ancient hot springs), is a place of pilgrimage for people from all parts of the world.

Many miracles have been achieved in answer to the famous cry of: "Rabbi Meir, save me!" Likewise cried the

Arab fishermen when suffering the lake storms, "'Rabbi Meir, save me!" For they all knew of the rabbi's miracles, and looked to him as the protector of all the lake fisherman, Arab or Jew.

I also called to Rabbi Meir once when, swimming foolishly far out across the lake, I was caught in a storm. Fierce gusts of wind had come – without reason or warning – down from the distant Golan peaks, turned red in a suddenly angry sky. The wind roared through the hill gullies and the lake waves were soon of a great height, the waters seething and flinging at the rocks along the shore, making return hazardous for any swimmer.

That time I experienced much difficulty in getting back to my children. They awaited me, with pale anxious faces, by the lakeside. They had been taught carefully by me, beside many seas, lakes and rivers of the world, never to enter deep water while I was out of reach of them. Nevertheless, as I struggled in the lake during that storm, I was possessed by the fear that if I did not return, one child after the other would go into the lake to seek for me, and that would be the end of us all.

Since experiencing that first Lake of Galilee storm as a swimmer, I was always very alert to any quickening of the lake breezes, and I would return at once to the shore. Shortly before my visit to Tiberias there had come a lake storm of hitherto unknown violence: certainly none of the oldest of fisherman remembered a storm of such power and danger. Many interpreted this as one more symptom of atomic bomb disruption, creating weather freaks in the remotest places of the world, vitiating the atmosphere of the universe.

In that storm many fishing-boats had been wrecked or damaged, and the lake itself had flung its waters at the town of Tiberias, pouring through the streets and flooding houses and doing much damage.

One Israeli friend had lost in the storm all of his carefully collected notes for a book on ancient Jewish and Arabian cookery, which he had gathered for many years, and would not have the patience to collect again, he told me. Therefore his book would never be completed.

Sometimes the Chamsin wind blew over the lake with molten fire in its breath, bringing dark whirling clouds of dust. Then one's lungs panted for cool air, and one prayed for the Chamsin to blow itself away; but it often blew for days.

Every day my children and I went to the lake to spend most of our hours there. I sat on the rocks, a distance out in the lake, doing my writing, and Rafik and Luz played around, in or out of the water. We lived by that lake over half a year; I could scarcely bear to be away from it for a day. When I went distances to Nazareth or Haifa, seldom returning before the evening, I yet went to the lake, often so late that the evening star was in the sky. The darkness and loneliness of the place then were compensated by the coolness of the water and the silver light upon the ripples.

Sometimes I reversed times, and before going on journeys would rise at dawn to bathe in the lake. The water was always very cool then, no matter how intense the heat had been. There could often be seen a milky moon still in the sky. It is that very hour by the lake which thus inspired a poet to praise:

> Abba! (*Father*) when the morn is breaking
> Through the portals of the sky,
> And the dappled fawns are waking
> In the reed-beds where they lie,
> And the milky moon looks mildly
> From the azure depths of heaven
> When the turtle doves are moaning
> In the rose isles where they lie.

The lake was always beautiful — every shifting, changing shade of it — at dawn, in the full sunlight, sunset or moonrise and full moon. The hills gave added interest to the water both as background and by their variety in reflection. They, burnt tawny as Bedouins from the many hot months of a Galilean summer, reflected their color in the lake. Then very often, for no reason at all other than the presence of currents, there were bars of the palest blue of chicory flowers reflected across the tawny expanses. This was especially usual along the Lebanon side. Also, facing the ruins of the old Jewish synagogue, with its old stone, age-worn landing-stage, there were usually to be seen dark, glassy areas, marking where the hot springs gushed into the lake, the dark places perfectly reflecting the old buildings of the south shore: up on the hillside the Rabbi Meir memorial and the baths of the hot springs.

The lake waters, when I saw them and swam in them from the beginning of summer to past its ending, were rarely the turquoise for which the Lake (Sea) of Galilee is famous. The heat was too white over the water most days, and the sky often almost colorless also: "the white-hot sky of Tiberias," of which many travelers have written. I recall mostly the grays and faint blues and the milky whites, like opals, and the rays of color striping the waters, rose, coral, amethyst, flax blue, fern green, or saffron. Sometimes the lake and its encircling hills were all one shade: a hyacinth blue matching the famed scented hyacinths of the Galil, which mist over the countryside in the early spring of Galilee.

Only the setting sun would put a brilliance on the summertime lake, making a broad path of fire, as the oranges of Jaffa for very color; and Rafik and Luz and their child friends of the lake shore, would pass to and fro along that path of orange light. Rafik swam along the pathway of the sun, for early in his fifth year he had learnt to swim well in the Lake of Galilee; Luz paddled or was taken swimming in my arms, or by friends. At sunset the kingfishers of the lake seemed stirred to increased activity, and the splashing of their diving was a continual sound of the evenings by the lake, as they launched themselves from the rocks or from the wreck of storm-torn eucalyptus boughs littered along the shingle.

Swallows also came lakewards in multitudes, and they companioned us as we swam, a delight to us always in their

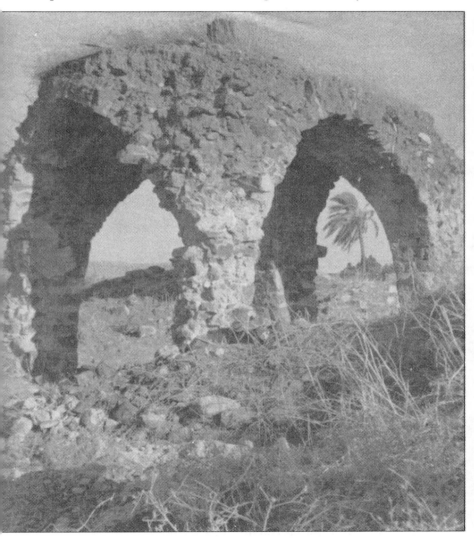

Old place by the Lake of Galilee

swiftness and grace of flashing wings. The swallows did not merely seek insects over the water, but refreshed themselves by dipping white breasts to red throats in the lake and sipping at the water.

Swallows are known to love clean water and are not found over dirty places. The Lake of Galilee has water which is sweet and limpid. The town of Tiberias is supplied with water from the lake. But, as many humans swim there, and also as some refuse of the town enters the lake, the drinking water in the taps has been heavily treated with chemical disinfectant, making it horrible to taste, and in my opinion, unnatural for the human body. There is big trade in soft drinks to disguise the unpleasant taste of modern Lake of Galilee water. I preferred to put crushed orange and lemon leaves, or jasmine flowers in our jugs of water.

Almost every day I would swim far out into the lake carrying a big jar with a screw-cap, to fill with pure, natural water from parts of the lake well beyond the area where it could be defiled by person or refuse. I would bring the jar back and my children would quench their thirst, and what was left I would carry back to our room. But water is a heavy thing to carry far, and the daily water-taking from the lake was always toilsome. I did this for my children because pure water is needed for making healthy blood and bone, and I think that mankind gives insufficient thought to the safeguarding of the natural purity of water. Therefore, when I return again to the Lake of Galilee I shall go to the area of Tagbha to stay, where there are many springs giving water which is a delight to drink for its purity and lightness.

The historic and beautiful River Jordan, which links the Sea of Galilee with the Dead Sea many miles away, was always a fascination and an interest to me when I lived above that river, years ago, in the north of Galilee.

I then made a home of a ruined Arab house in a deserted and destroyed Arab village, my big Afghan hound with me as a guard. From that house I could see the River Jordan passing not far away below, in its coiling beauty. But to go down to that river had been forbidden, because there the Jordan divided Israel from Syria, and it could easily be waded from either shore, and therefore the land on the Israel side had been heavily mined.

But despite the unpleasant thought of the mines, I knew that I could not leave Galilee without having bathed in the Jordan which had daily tempted me whenever I looked down on it. On very calm days of great heat, it had been possible to hear the clamor of those swift-flowing waters from my house above. To have lived close by the Jordan River and never to have bathed in it was to fail in experience of life: It was to be a baptism for me!

I had to go there alone because the visit was forbidden to all; nor could I risk endangering my dog with the mines planted in that area. I had taken a long branch of eucalyptus tree with me to beat a path ahead of me and search for mines. The steep descent to the river below was quite easy walking for the first quarter mile because it led to one of the kibbutz water tanks, but from there on I met with a wilderness of rocks set around with thistles and thorns which scratched at my legs and arms and cut my sandals. It was snakeland there also, for numerous times I heard the rustle of snake bodies hastening away at the sound of my coming.

When I arrived within sight of the rich verdure spreading out for some distance on either side of the river, that green beauty in its surrounding of sun-scorched brown scrub urged me onward despite the increasing difficulties and the true pain of the descent. I wanted some of the scented oleander blossoms of the Jordan, and to see the hummingbirds, about which I had been told.

Then, when the sound of the river came clearly to me —

a rushing torrent of water by the sound of it – I was halted by a fear greater than that of mines or snakes. On a hill exactly facing the path where I was beating my way to the river, and where I had planned to bathe, I made out the forms of three men watching me from their Syrian territory, and all three seemed to be pointing guns towards my path.

I took a long time then trying to decide whether or not I dared risk a quick dash down to the river for my bath, if I could get there and then back up the hillside before I was within range of gunfire. I decided to go onwards to the Jordan. My decision proved a good one. For as I had approached closer to the Syrian hills, I found that the three men with pointing guns were in reality only tall thorn bushes! I held out my arms to them then, and laughed, and went onwards to the river joyfully, thankful that fear had not deprived me of the beauty which was beginning to reveal itself in water flashing through green places.

When I arrived at the very river, the scene there was unforgettable. The earth blossomed! Oleanders grew in scented thickets and mingled their white or red flowers with the intense yellow blooms of carob trees which pressed against them. There were the silver willows of Galilee of the singing leaves, sweet perfumed purple buddleia, hawthorn, and arbutus bushes, wild figs and vines, and along the water edge a variety of wild mints and cresses which gave out pungent scents as I stepped upon them, to enter – at last! – the River Jordan which had tormented and enticed me for over a month, as it flowed away below my house.

I seemed to have entered a different land, the contrast was so great: from the thorny parched waste with its company of snakes that I had left only minutes ago, to the present lushness and fragrance, where wild bees thronged and hummingbirds hovered amongst massed blossoms.

I took off my clothes and entered the waters of the Jordan. Where I bathed the river was quite shallow, no more than thigh deep, but the force of the rushing waters made it necessary for me to cling to overhanging oleander boughs as I crossed the river to walk on Syrian earth. I would have been swept down the river otherwise. I was pleased to know the sort of water which fed the Lake of Galilee, and on my return to the lake years later, whenever I saw oleander blossoms floating on its waters I would imagine that they had come down from the Jordan.

I took my children to look upon that river from a hillside in northern Galilee. Times were no more peaceful between Israel and Syria than they had been during my other visit, and I felt that the mines would yet be there down the hillsides, therefore we had to be content with merely looking from a distance at the historic river.

I told Rafik and Luz about the three trees which had resembled Syrian rifleman, and we laughed about that. I showed my children the Huleh Lake and its surrounding wild marshland, now considerably drained and planted with crops. The haunts of the big white pelicans were once there, and I remembered the body of one of those great birds which I had seen nailed to the wall of the dining room of the Turkish kibbutz in northern Galilee. The wings of that bird had spanned over eight feet. It had been shot when taking fish from the kibbutz ponds. The pelican had been dead when nailed, but there on the wall in its pure white majesty it had looked crucified to me.

The three-mile long triangular Lake Huleh is a sister lake to Galilee. In former days the Arabs called it the "Wheat Sea" because of the far-stretching areas of wheat cultivated in the surrounding marshes. There is also a region of wild yellow, sometimes white, water lilies which transform into loveliness the muddy waters of Huleh Lake and swamp.

Once water buffalo were to be found in those swamps and in areas around the Lake of Galilee. In river and lakeside caves in Galilee ancient remains of rhinoceros have been discovered, as has one immense elephant skeleton, thought to be one of the army elephants of Genghis Khan run amok.

Once, in many places along the shores of the Jordan, groves of the sacred terebinth trees were to be found, and the terebinth is yet often seen in Galilee. Believers went there for cure of diseases, or to leave in the care of the "spirit of the grove" their bundles of papyrus reeds cut from the swamp, from which they would make quantities of mats, and even small houses, especially temporary lakeside houses for the fishermen. The people knew that no thief would dare to violate the terebinth shrines or to take anything left in their custody.

Near Caesarea, by the lake, there was once a shrine to the god Pan where icy water gushes out from hard rock, typical of the spring-fed torrents of Galilee which are such a joy to travelers, who plunge dusty sunburnt faces and arms and legs into the ice of those torrents: that is a reason to worship water!

Onwards, beyond Galilee, the River Jordan drains itself away into the Dead Sea, into those mysterious waters of death which stretch far into the southern desert.

In our months by the lake we chose rocks on both shores, north and south, for our own almost daily use, because, as all were in distant places, no one else ever wanted them. Only when we were in a hurry, going away from the lake on an exploration somewhere, did we bathe close by the town. The water was clean enough there on the south side, but I could not bear to swim and have my eyes on the tombs in the Jewish and Arab cemeteries which face the lake on low foothills. Surely, as I said before, few cemeteries are so close to water, and such historic water.

It is also a piece of land known for its wild flowers: the purple iris and knee-tall daffodils, whilst a short distance above the cemetery on King Herod's Castle Hill grow the golden flowers first described in Homer's verse, which tell of the meadows of Hades clothed with the golden flowers, asphodels, said to be the food for the dead. Their starchy roots are yet eaten by peasants in eastern countries, including Palestine and Arabia. They are usually mixed with the sweeter roots of the mallows, and then make a nutritious food with a nutty taste. I have eaten them in Gypsy homes in Istanbul.

Castle Hill and the foothills of the cemetery are also the territory of purple anemones, which mass there, and scented wild cyclamens of many colors, shading from ivory to rose like the flesh of young women. To be buried by the Lake of Galilee! All that water, and the wild flowers, and teeming birds! The dead in their graves . . . how is it for them when the iris cover the cemetery of Tiberias with their purple groves of sweet-scented flowers early every spring, or when the jackals come prowling in the night, thrusting their pointed snouts into the earth where it has been newly turned? What can the dead experience of all that?

The ancients cried to their children: "Ye are blood of my blood, bone of my bone." That truth expects that, through all the generations, humans see and enjoy places and things of the earth again through their children because they continue to live on in their children: the same blood, the same bone. I could see and hear my own son and daughter observing and commenting on Galilee in a way similar to myself. Yet about death no one can be sure. For with all our human cleverness – often a terrible cleverness, as in modern times when we bombard the very heavens – death yet remains the mystery of mysteries.

I think that Colette, the French writer, had a good plan for herself to remain on the earth after death. She said that because of her love for travel, her skin should be made into a small trunk so that part of herself would continue to travel. It seems to me a plan to copy!

Relics found along Galilee's southern shore tell of the great age of the lake: There are to be seen remains of massive granite pillars which indicate what might have been once a long colonnaded avenue of shade along the lake border, where the pagan people of King Herod Antipas's ill-famed city had sought protection from the blaze of the Tiberian sunlight. The pillars also were to be found away from the lake, in the fields beyond. There some of them yet stand upright; others lean forwards or backwards at tottering angles, one supporting another, and wild pigeons from their dens in the hill caves above, where they live in multitudes, perch in amorous pairs upon the ancient columns.

The column bases, worn down to wide flat circles, extend most of the way along the southern shore to below the hot springs, and these made a game of stepping stones for my children.

All of the half year and more that we lived in Tiberias we passed our days in the way of nomads, out of doors from early morning to sunset, even to starlight, wandering by the lake. We passed many hours merely basking like seals on the rocks, so that our flesh became the very color of Gypsy copperware.

The north shore provided an interesting pastime because there were hillocks of clay seemingly thrown up by the water turtles, certainly by some creature, the clay texture being very fine, similar to that of molehills. This made excellent modeling material when mixed with the lake water, and we made numerous things: little basins and cups and dishes, toy animals, boats and houses. We decorated many of the clay objects with brightly colored small stones found amongst the shingle. We used a flat rock on which to sun-bake our clay; it required two days of sunlight to achieve a hard-enough bake so that the toys could be carried on the long walk back to our garden without fear of breakage. There they were enjoyed in daily play or presented to the child friends of Rafik and Luz.

My children often swapped their clay things for dom fruits or dates, to which better tree-climbers had better access, although, by the lake, quantities of dom fruits could be obtained merely by strongly shaking the branches.

As we were frequent visitors to the same places north and south along the lake, and made very little noise when there (as my children from an early age had known that to play as quietly as the wild animals themselves was to share places with many of them), we had for company numerous birds, fish, and some water turtles. The shy kingfishers and ice birds soon accepted our presence and dived for fish from rocks within close reach of us, as unconcernedly as if we ourselves had been three rocks. The fish came to know us for they fed on the pips from the melons that we ate most days, and the peel of oranges; also the residue from the quantities of maize [corn] which we ate raw. They knew our eating times, our early morning meal of fruit, and our bigger meal at midday when we had the maize and cos lettuce, and the salty white cheese from ewe's milk, also with pita bread, the big wheel-shaped loaves of flour not brown enough to really please us, but at least not of lifeless white flour.

The lake fish became very tame. I have heard of carp being tamed, coming to a calling human voice, or to a whistle blown. Many Chinese legends tell of princesses who possessed tame goldfish or carp. Although carp like to live in cold water, there are carp in the Lake of Galilee, also barbell and catfish, locally called *barbut* from a colloquial Arab word for splashing. And splash they do, adding their part to the music of the lake. There are also sardines in quantity.

The Spanish mystic, St. John of the Cross, petted the fish of Granada's rivers, Genil and Darro. He would call to the friars accompanying him: "Come here, brothers, and see how these little creatures of God are praising him as they swim to and fro."

Summer in Galilee

We tamed one large fish to which we gave the Turkish name of *gunesh*, meaning the sun. That species of fish was beautiful, but was of a kind I did not know, being patterned in the manner of a fritillary flower in a faint checkered way, with its fins and tail of sunlight yellow, and yellow patches over its eyes. It was a big fish to be seen close to the shore. Gunesh soon came to take slices of bread from our fingers and let us stroke his back as he fed with us. We also fed grains of maize to him and pieces of pomegranate. He appeared to be a fish of importance, for when he flashed his round golden eyes and flicked his saffron tail, all the lesser fish fled to a distance. He liked to dine alone.

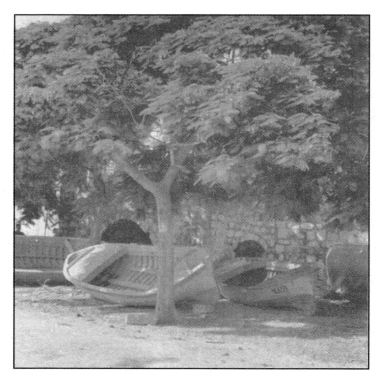

Boats beneath pepper trees: Tiberias

Only, having tamed the fish, we suffered misgivings that our Gunesh might be taken by one of the lakeside fishermen, that for our own selfish pleasure we had probably endangered the fish's life. However, the months went by and no fishermen came with their quivering rods or their flinging nets to disturb our peace. That place seemed too rocky to encourage them. Only once did we meet a fisherman there, and on my asking him fearfully to show us what he had caught, he told us that he had taken nothing: a big fish with yellow fins and tail had carried off the bait from his line but had not been taken itself! We felt after having the fisherman's information that we could leave the Lake of Galilee with minds more tranquil, for our tamed Gunesh was cleverer, and therefore more safe, than we had believed.

Now I think the crabs of the Lake of Galilee illustrated the colored variety of the waters better even than the beautiful flashing kingfishers of both species, the lesser and the great. The Galilee crabs scurried out from their tunnel houses beneath the rocks in the shallows, not in the usual drab crab tones of fawn or gray or near black; they came in the colors of the anemones of the Galil. In purple and rose and light green they appeared, freckled with gold or silver, streaked with amber, smudged with indigo. And as the crabs hastened through the water shallows, they disturbed from concealed places (and thus revealed to us beachcombers by the lake) diminutive square pieces of mosaic of several colors, and of age equal to that of Tiberias itself, for they had come from the walls of King Herod's palace where they had once made decorations in the form of great and monstrous animals.

From our first discovery of the pieces of mosaic — tiny cubes of brilliant shade of greens, blues, and some yellows — we searched for them daily. "Rock," Rafik and Luz called the little pieces, and between them found so many (because their seeking was endless) that, added to my own findings, we possessed nearly one hundred before we left Tiberias.

Summer in Galilee

Some had the texture and color of cubes of jade, others of the blue lapis lazuli or very hard glass; the yellow seemed to be made from sulfurous rock. There were no other colors to be found, though those three primary colors were in all shades.

Animal images were forbidden by the laws of Moses and therefore, history relates, the mosaics of King Herod's palace had given offense to the religious Jews within sight of Tiberias since their first hour of existence. They must have been very conspicuous from far off, especially when struck by the noon sunlight which bathes Castle Hill until sunset, or they would not have given deep provocation to the religious Jews which finally resulted in Herod's great palace being attacked and the mosaics scattered from the hillside on which stood the palace.

That had been done under the cover of the Roman-Jewish wars. Now, nearly two thousand years after, the mosaic pieces were yet being pushed up by the crabs of the Lake of Galilee, or washed free of the concealing shingle by the lake waves, especially in times of storm; also when modern irrigation causes the lake to recede far back from its normal boundaries. The pieces which we found were notably of conspicuous colorings and glittered most beautifully, especially when dipped in the lake to remove the dullness caused by great age.

It had certainly been a Jewish religious mob, not any organized Roman army, which had destroyed the palace of Herod during that time when it had become the property of Herod Agrippa's son. The complete destruction took place between the years 66–70 A.D.

The Herod Antipas who had built the place and also built Tiberias, was the sovereign of Christ. His father was Herod the Great who, as the New Testament tells, commanded that all the children of Bethlehem under the age of two years should be slain. The son, called merely Herod in the Bible, was the Tetrarch of Galilee and Perea, whose second wife was Herodius, and it was he who had John the Baptist beheaded.

When the sweet waters of the Lake of Galilee are used for irrigation, crops and trees of all kinds can be grown. There are also the dew clouds which fall over the mountains of Galilee. This dew, *tal* in the Bible, is really the product of clouds which have blown down from the north, from Mount Hermon, which dominates the mountains of Galilee, and which settles on the highlands when the sun has set. The rising lake mists also deposit dew by night.

On the wide plain of Gennesaret by the lake are grown maize, melons, marrows [summer squash, zucchini], tomatoes, peppers, eggplant, and ladies' fingers or bamiyeh (*Hibiscus esculentis*), a delicious-tasting small vegetable looking more like green Chinese lanterns than ladies' fingers; also grapes and bananas, and then further, tobacco.

On the foothills there are fig and pomegranate trees everywhere, also mulberries, walnuts, almonds, apricots, peaches, and pears. Apples are a specialty of the Galil, especially in the north, and orange and lemon trees scent the air along many a stretch of the lake shore, and are found in most of the old gardens in Tiberias.

On the higher hills, and also in the Jordan valley, wild medicinal herbs are plentiful. The aromatic ones such as rosemary, marjoram, and many kinds of thyme, scent the air most pleasantly, and are valuable for the essential oils that they yield. Fennel grows everywhere by the lake and on the hills far up into the highest ranges of upper Galilee. In green Lilliputian forests the fennel grows, giving salad food for man and abundant nourishment for animals, especially the goats who greatly love that plant. The Romans ate fennel for the principal purpose of quickening their minds and improving their memory. Soldiers of all periods, including the Crusaders when in the Holy Land, have eaten fennel to give them courage in battle.

Olive trees are very plentiful, and concerning the olive trees of Galilee, the Talmud says that "It is easier to raise a legion of olive trees in Galilee than one child in Judaea." This statement was influenced by the former plagues which carried off Jewish children in great numbers.

When we lived close by the lake, my own children suffered from a skin ailment, very common in the old town of Tiberias, but less prevalent in the new town on the hillside. This ailment seemed to be very contagious and when my own children had this and therefore I became aware of it, I noticed the infection frequently on the faces and limbs of other children, Jewish and Arab.

The common name for the ailment was furuncles, and the malady seemed to be a form of fungus similar to ringworm. Great deep pits appear in the skin, and over them form thick and numerous scabs which scale off. Newcomers to the lower regions of Galilee are more likely to be infected, as copious sweating opens the pores and softens the flesh unduly. I spoke with Mrs. Yaccub, a pharmacist from Baghdad, who told me that her children had never been free of the ailment after coming to Tiberias, despite countless dollars having been spent on the best modern medicinal treatments, including penicillin. She blamed the old town for the infection, as when she took her children to live in a new, modern suburb of Tiberias, the ailment was soon overcome.

Being an herbalist myself, and having written several books on herbal medicine, I chose natural substances for the cure of my own children. Certainly penicillin is of purely vegetable origin, but in modern medicine the primary wish seems to be to try to improve upon nature, the "improving" often being done from commercial interests. Much of the healing power of penicillin has been lost already, and when the molds of penicillin have been highly processed, or made in a synthetic form, the remedy can prove harmful, especially when given as an injection for internal treatment.

The Bible promised herbs for the healing of humans, and that was good enough for my children and me: Herbs, pure and always marvelous in their deep and unchanging healing powers, have never failed me.

For my medicines I chose two natural things: the fruits of the lemon tree for external and internal use, and clay from the Lake of Galilee to use as an external healer. I had read in one of Edmond Bordeaux Szekely's books that Saint John, who more than any other of the disciples of Christ inherited His healing powers and practiced natural medicine, used clay from the Lake of Galilee to heal skin diseases, leprosy, and severe infections of the bones. Now I was given reason to test the curative powers of that clay.

It was remarkable how fast, within a few days, the infection spread. I had imagined, when I saw the first sores on my children's skin, that the eruptions were bites from the lake flies. It was impossible to protect against the lake flies with the herbal lotion which I used effectively against mosquitoes every night, because my children and I were in and out of the water the day through, and any lotion would soon be washed away and was too expensive to waste in that manner. I had never been warned about the furuncles and had taken no precautions.

Rafik's entire chin was infected, also his nostrils deep within, and of Luz, one entire leg from heel to thigh, and also her nostrils. I had only slight ailment, because my skin had been well hardened by many years of life under a blazing sun, so that it was as toughened and hardened as that of any old nomad Gypsy. I had a sore above my upper lip and one on the far side of my face, and, as with my children, my nostrils were infected.

I was pleased to have those many lemon trees in the garden of the house in old Tiberias; fruits were heavy on the boughs where they would remain until the Succoth festival at summer's ending when full autumn came. Lemons are highly antiseptic and revitalize the blood. My children shared the juice of one every morning, even when in full health. How sweet are those lemons of Galilee, ripened in that abundant sunlight, and how good is such clean natural medicine.

Clay was obtainable in quantities from the lake, especially along the north shore. There the turtles or terrapins were a help to me because they made big heaps of fine clay, and when I further sifted this through a wire strainer to remove grit and small pebbles, it was ready for mixing with the lake water into a paste to be applied to our skin.

My little girl Luz had an entire clay-covered left leg, but she did not mind. I felt on my own face the powerful drawing properties of the clay; it seemed to possess special dynamic qualities. After only one week of clay treatments combined with use of lemon juice, my sores were all healed, and my children were on the way to being healed. My herbal treatments, especially the use of the lake clay, was much criticized by the people of Tiberias, and I was daily rebuked for not taking my children to a doctor, and was further told repeatedly that natural treatments could not possibly cure such a serious ailment.

The raw lemon juice lotion had to be applied during the late night when Rafik and Luz were in their deepest hours of sleep, in order that they should not feel its smarting action, as it attacked the infection, whereas the clay treatment was given during the day, and it was often necessary for my children to walk back from the lake with their skin plastered with clay. But as the treatment was proving so effective we did not mind the amusement that we caused, and were indeed amused ourselves.

Then, when we were all completely cured — while others using orthodox chemicals and ointments and penicillin made little progress at all — our critics praised our clean, healed flesh. But they still considered it too eccentric to use clay in this modern age of advanced medicine! And also it was too troublesome! However, if some Israeli pharmacy firm under supervision of the Government would market the clay of the Lake of Galilee, and not spoil it by any refining treatment, they would be doing a great service to sick humanity.

It was of deep interest to me to be using a treatment which had been successful in the days of Christ, nearly two thousand years ago. It is known that from the shores of that strange Lake of Galilee, many hundreds of feet below sea-level, Christ gathered almost exclusively His earliest disciples, all destined to be famous whilst the world lasts. It was the Crusaders who brought back to Europe from the Holy Land evidence that Christ's favorite disciples, John and James, came from Tiberias; and this was later carefully confirmed by the historian Petrus Diaconus, whose writings time has proved to be remarkably correct.

In Galilee, and especially near the lake, I thought much about Christ. He had been a Galilean, Jesus of Galilee the people called him, and an orthodox Jew, celebrating there the various Jewish festivals, preaching in the synagogues, Himself shepherding in the hills, bathing in the lake, which He, together with the great rabbis who had come there also, have made the most holy water on earth.

Surely the especial loveliness of Galilee was the reason why God chose Nazareth for the boyhood of Jesus, and the Lake of Galilee environs for most of Christ's manhood.

Once I had seen a party of young Italian women, all of them beautiful, accompanied by a Franciscan priest in brown habit, kneeling on a part of the north shore which reaches out into the Lake of Galilee, singing there as sweet-voiced as a charm of nightingales. When I asked them about their visit they said they had come to the lake to sing for Christ.

Beautiful things made me wonder: Did He see this very beauty? Had He eaten dom fruits and enjoyed the pungent scent of the wild buddleia by the lake, the beauty of the shore birds, butterflies, dragonflies, and lizards?

On the hillside behind where we gathered the clay, there bloomed wild tulips in the early spring, half as high as Rafik and red as dragon's blood. It appeared that they had always grown there, propagating themselves through the centuries by seed and bulb. Had He seen them growing? Had the Crusaders plucked them to wear tucked in their armor when they rode out on their many known sallies from Tiberias to war against the Saracens and to die, most of them, on the plains or amongst the hills of Galilee?

❧

There were unpleasant things to mar the beauty of the life of the Lake of Galilee: the meanness or the stupidity of man, and the molestation of the biting insects frequently spoilt the pleasure of the lake.

Pickpockets lurked in the shadow of trees and bushes to prey on bathers in the lake. My purse was picked of nearly five pounds at a time when I was very short of money and could ill spare a penny! I never thought of pickpockets by a holy lake, and had never taken precautions. That money had been with me when bathing because I was traveling onwards to Haifa. I was swimming too far from the shore to return immediately when I saw a young man run to the eucalyptus tree where I had hung the basket holding my clothes and purse. I was thankful that the thief never found my old Tunisian silver earrings which I had taken out of my ears while swimming, and which also had been in the basket.

The police seemed little interested when I reported my loss to them. Friends told me later that such thefts were commonplace, and people who knew Tiberias better than I never took anything of value to the lake. Will it be necessary one day to nail boards to the trees along the shore of the holy lake, inscribed with the warning "Beware of Pickpockets!"?

Then, the orthodox young men were often a nuisance to women and girl children in the matter of lake bathing. Those young men apparently are taught to look upon female creatures as unclean and are taught not bathe close to them. That is well enough – all can have their special beliefs – only orthodox young men should have their own fenced-off bathing area! As it is, they bathed anywhere and then considered that they had the pious right to stone women and children who bathe in the lake near to them. They certainly stoned Luz and me.

In Tiberias the orthodox are now very numerous, as this city is a holy one of the Jews ever since the great Rabbi Ben Yochai removed the curse of uncleanness from Tiberias, under which stigma it suffered in its early years during the time of Christ. During the time of Ben Yochai the seat of the great Jewish patriarch and the Sanhedrin was transferred to Tiberias, and it remains one of the miracles of Jewish history that the once unclean capital of Herod Antipas, pagan and disreputable, should become the new Jerusalem of the Jews and the home of many of Judaism's greatest rabbis and sages.

Tiberias became then, and continues to be, a holy city and a place of authority for all the dispersed Jewish communities of the world. It is a further strange fact that Tiberias on the Lake of Galilee, where Christianity had much of its origin, is a center of Jewish theology, and the colleges of the great rabbis, established there centuries ago, still exist to this day, flourishing and powerful, and attracting disciples from all parts of the world, but especially from the Jewish Ashkenazi (Eastern European) sect.

The orthodox young men keep their heads covered to demonstrate their sanctity, and wear round, cotton caps even as they bathe in the lake. They all grow ear-locks, which are kept generally carefully oiled and curled. They keep themselves apart from all women with the exception of their own mothers if they live at home during any period of their studies.

My first awareness of their belief in the uncleanness of women and girls was when Luz and I were stoned as we bathed in the Lake of Galilee. The leader of that particular band of youths was a fat young man whom I had often noticed on the bus for Kiryat Samuel. He had attracted my attention, not through reasons of his fatness, but from his theatrical and unctuous air, and the way that he kept firmly to his bus seat, always leaving women, old as well as young, standing beside the seat which he occupied. I had also marveled at the tallow whiteness of his flesh in Tiberias of the endless sunlight.

I sent my frightened children out of the lake, but I continued to swim, although all of the time I was puzzled by such a demonstration.

When I saw Moise, a friend from Egypt, swimming towards me, I asked the reason for the stones and the ugly cries coming from the young men. He told me of their belief that women, and even girl children, contaminated water and therefore they did not want them to bathe in close proximity.

I then told Moise that it was absurd; we were beyond stone-throw of the youths and the lake was deep and wide. Surely we *were* beyond stone-throw, for none of the missiles had touched me or my children. I said also that the orthodox youths themselves must go farther away if they wished to demonstrate their righteousness! Moise swam away to tell the youths what I said. They continued to bathe and I continued to bathe! Then, as they left the water before me, and as they passed by within reach of my voice, I told them in Hebrew:

"Next time you go away; you! You! You!"

"No, you! You! You!" they flung back at me.

Afterwards, when lack of time caused me to have to bathe close by the town where we might meet with the orthodox young men, and I was in the water already when they came by, I always shouted at them: "You! You! You!" and they knew what I meant and went farther along the shore. But if they were bathing when I arrived by the lake, I then went well away with my children; and therefore there was no more trouble between us concerning lake bathing.

The biting flies of the lake were a molestation; except in the very remote places, they were usually there seeking human blood. There were little gray flies of common house-fly form, very silent, pricking one's flesh most of the time when one was out of the water; also a flat fly with spotted body and also flat wings barred with yellow. Their bite was more painful. Sometimes the really big ones came, the type which preyed on the mules and donkeys, but were not impartial to human blood. I am sure that my children and I, being vegetarians like those animals on which the big flies preyed, received more than our normal share of such bites! We protected ourselves very well against mosquitoes by night with the use of herbs, but, as I have written, it was hopeless to protect against the lake flies when our bodies were constantly dripping with the lake water.

The disadvantages of the lakeside life were small compared with the beauty which met the eyes on all sides. When the Lake of Galilee lay like a stretch of eastern silk, shade of the gray herons of the lake, barred with fruit-blossom colors and with threads of silver and gold from the reflected light and the encircling hills, and we could bask like seals stretched out on the dark rocks, those old and historical rocks, the fire of the sun putting a pleasing torpor on our flesh and dazzling our eyes when raised towards it — then the life of the lake was only pleasant. The flies then could be endured, and the beauty yet enjoyed as humans of all kinds have gloried in it through the ages, and will continue to while the Lake of Galilee exists.

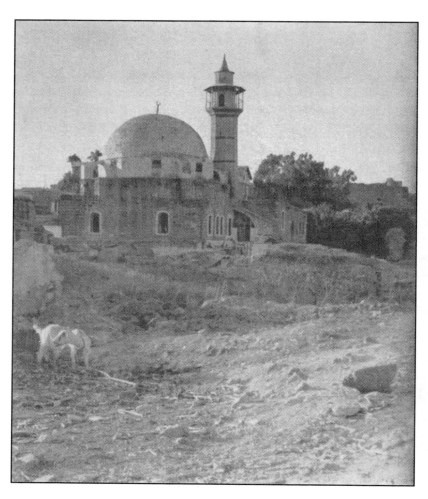

Old Tiberias

Chapter Three

Life in Tiberias

Modern Tiberias occupies only a small area of the great Roman city founded by King Herod Antipas. The wide boundaries of the old walls can still be traced.

The town began its existence as an unclean city, because – in order that it should be built by the shore of the Lake of Galilee, on the best site for fine views and coolness and easy access to the famous hot springs – corpses had to be removed from the old cemetery which reached so close to the borders of the lake that its waters lapped over many tombstones. Ancient Jewish law forbids the removal of corpses, and curses as unclean all places where this law had been trespassed against. The lake city therefore was considered unclean by the Jews, and no religious Jew would approach near to the place. Therefore King Herod had to open the jails to populate his city, and had to bring slaves to occupy the grand houses that he had built; riffraff from other lands and their "fancy women" came also to settle there.

In his classic book, *Jewish Antiquities*, Flavius Josephus, great historian of the Jews and also a leader in the Roman-Jewish wars, gives an account of how Tiberias was built:

> And now Herod the Tetrarch who was in great favor with Tiberias, built a city of the same name within Galilee, at the Lake of Gennesaret. There are warm

baths at a little distance from it, in a village named Ammaus. Strangers came and inhabited the city; a great number of the inhabitants were Galileans, also many were caused by Herod to come thither out of the country belonging to him, and were by force compelled to be its inhabitants. Some of them were persons of condition. He also admitted poor people, such as those who were collected from all parts to dwell in it; in fact, some of them were not quite free men, and to them he was a benefactor and made them free in great numbers, but he obliged them not to forsake the city by building them very good houses at his own expense and by giving them land also.

This lakeside city was therefore considered as unclean for years, and further a pagan place of ill repute. It is much disputed whether or not Christ ever entered Tiberias. It was not until a century and a half after the building of the town that it was miraculously made clean by the great Rabbi Ben Yochai, who had been a principal disciple of the yet greater Rabbi Akiba, "The Martyr," both of them rabbis of Galilee.

Ben Yochai, when his life was considered past saving from an incurable disease, entered the unclean city to bathe in the hot springs of Tiberias in the Roman baths there, and was immediately cured of the illness. He interpreted his cure as a sign from God, and, showing great moral courage, he then, ignoring great hostility, pronounced Tiberias clean.

But that was over a century after the crucifying of Christ, and as Christ came from a very religious orthodox Jewish family, it is said that He would not have dared to enter the unclean Tiberias. Then, again, it is argued that as He went fearlessly where humanity most needed reform, Tiberias was the very place to have attracted His help. Then further there were several synagogues in Tiberias even during its period of uncleanness, and the Bible clearly states of Christ that He preached in "all the synagogues of Galilee." Nowhere is it written "in all the synagogues excepting those of Tiberias."

And His close disciples, John and James, are known to have come from Tiberias. No one can be sure concerning Christ and Tiberias. I feel that He went there; others — far better qualified to form an opinion — believe likewise.

The hot springs of Tiberias have been famous from time immemorial. Julius Caesar is known to have bathed there. He was a naturalist, and I have a special sympathy for him on one count because he once said that he owed his great health to the use of honey within and oil without, and I can nearly say the same; but sympathy with little else concerning that ruthless Roman conqueror. He would have loved the honey of Galilee with its rich scent and flavor of aromatic mountain flowers and tree blossoms.

The hot springs have survived the fall of Greece and Rome, the rise and quick decline of the Crusaders, followed by Mamluks and Turks. Now, after the end of the British occupation, they are being greatly enlarged by the Israelis.

The present baths were built in the middle of the nineteenth century by Ibrahim Pasha during the Egyptian occupation of Palestine, and improvements were then made by the following Turkish government, the baths possessing a very oriental type of outer architecture, although within they remain distinctly Roman.

The temperature of the springs is nearly 140° F. The waters contain numerous minerals and also [safe] radioactive properties. They are considered to resemble the waters of Carlsbad in many ways, cures for rheumatism, skin diseases, and bone infections being reported. The hot springs have beautiful and cool hillside gardens, with shady date palms and groves of pines where the sick are refreshed by natural beauty and the cool breezes rising from the Lake of Galilee close below.

The buildings of the hot springs and baths are neighbor to the memorial tomb of Rabbi Meir (see photo, page 111) and look towards the ruins of the ancient lakeside synagogue.

Summer in Galilee

In times of national peril, including the recent Sinai war, the *shofar*, a ram's horn trumpet, is heard being blown mysteriously from the synagogue ruins, and no living man is the trumpeter. People have said that they have heard it; they say how it enters into the heart.

The Jewish *shofar* is made from the horn of a large ram, and is blown especially at the ending of the Jewish Fast of Yom Kippur, when neither food nor drink may be taken throughout one entire night and the following day. Such fasting is not difficult in temperate climates, but a night and day without drink in the late summer heat of Tiberias is an ordeal. I know this, for I kept the Fast of Yom Kippur when in Tiberias.

During the many times that Tiberias has been attacked, large numbers of the population have gone into hiding in the subterranean passages which go from the city deep into Castle Hill of King Herod's palace – or once went there. The caves on the hillside stretching much of the way to the hot springs were also hiding places for the Tiberians: their height and the rocky ways to them giving security to the dwellers within. They have also been much used by hermits and robbers. Sulfurous fumes belch out from many caves, making them seem witch-like and strange.

I searched for, though never discovered, the underground places; but I did visit with my children one evening the caves overlooking the southern shore of the lake. We climbed towards the setting sun, and our arrival at the first of the numerous caverns was greeted by a mob of wild pigeons, which came together like a gray smoke-cloud, rising and falling above us, only with such a music of whirring wings as is not known to silent smoke. Hundreds upon hundreds of pigeons veered out from the caves and I wondered on what they lived, with the land for a distance all around them being parched into brown wastes by the summer sun.

There were dom trees with their almost perpetual fruiting on the hillsides, and some dates left on the highest branches of the palms, out of reach up there of the thrown stones of the water-side boys who were expert in stoning fruit off trees. There was little more. Indeed the only green things to be seen, apart from the nonedible lakeside shrubs and trees, were melon seedlings which had grown up from the pips dropped by melon-eaters on the lake shore.

Apart from the emerging pigeons, there was nothing to see in those Galilean caves. But there was atmosphere about them of great age, and a brooding strangeness which made us hasten away before the quick dusk of Galilee left us there in the darkness. When we were only a short distance away down the steep path a loud knocking came from one of the highest caverns of all. That was quite frightening, for there was the beat of human motion in the knocking, and we were so far away from friendly people. Back in Tiberias, I was told that no one should go to the caves alone, and that they had an evil reputation.

Crusaders are said to have used those caves to stable their horses. That was of interest to me. As I was reading, for much of my time in Tiberias, Villehardouin's *Chronicle* and Joinville's *Memoir of the Crusades*, all concerning the Crusaders – or their horses – was of interest to me. Often, around the old places, I imagined that I could hear the rattle of the chain armor which the knights had worn in battle despite its unsuitable nature in a climate of great heat, and hear also the stamping feet of their big war horses from Europe, as out of place as the armor for use on sandy plains or rocky hills, and all having a need for much water.

Those splendid horses from England, France, and Italy had arrived in the Holy Land sick from the long sea voyages, where they mostly had traveled in the holds of the ships, as it is written:

> On the day that we entered into our ship from
> Marseilles in August, we opened the hold door and

led in our horses, and then caulked the door well, as when a cask is sunk in water, because when the ship is on the high sea all the said door is under water.

It can well be understood that horses so transported would later stand a poor chance in combat against the hardy ponies and camels of the Saracen Saladin and others, against whom the Crusaders warred with valor, but with short-lasting success. The Crusaders in that furnace heat of Galilee – and especially when in Tiberias, those hundreds of feet below sea level – longed for the cool airs of their lands in Europe, and there is a pathetic description in the *Memoir of the Crusades* indicating the nostalgia of the knights for cool meres and their swans, when telling of the coming of the Prince of Antioch:

> With him came three gentlemen from Armenia, going on pilgrimage to Jerusalem, and they had three horns, so devised that the sound came from the side of their faces. When they began to sound their horns you would had said it was the voice of swans coming from a mere, for they made the sweetest music and the most melodious.

As for the dysentery which afflicted the Crusaders and weakened them greatly (and is yet a common malady in Galilee, especially for new-comers) the *Memoir* told:

> The Knights and King Lewis of France himself, had to have the lower parts of their drawers cut away because of the severe dysentery from which they suffered and so frequent their necessities.

The circuit of the Lake of Galilee in the New Testament times included many peoples antagonistic one to another.

Tiberias, the great Roman city, despite its ill repute, was for a time the capital of that area, and was close to the Greek cities of Gadara and Hippos, all intensely anti-Jewish and similarly hated by the Jews. There was Taricheai and Gamala, where terrible massacres occurred in the Jewish risings against the Romans. Indeed all around the lake, history relates the cries of wars, of conquerors and their victims; and in times of peace, other cries, the incantations of the people sacrificing to heathen gods within the groves. It was in such an atmosphere that Christ came to preach peace.

Although it was in Galilee that the Christian church had its origin, Christianity has always suffered a perilous existence there. In the early centuries of Christianity there came the rise of the powerful rabbinism in Tiberias and Safed; later, when Christianity did become the religion of the district, its survival was short, for corruption within enabled the Arab prophet Mohammed to come forth in the seventh century and replace Christianity throughout Galilee and far beyond.

A few centuries later, the militant Christianity of the Crusaders arrived and was crushed out of existence in one of the crudest massacres of world history, at the battle of the Horns of Hattin, along the north region of the Lake of Galilee between Tiberias and Nazareth.

Since then, Christianity has only really flourished amongst the small communities of monks and nuns living within or beyond Tiberias, especially now in Nazareth. Not far beyond Tiberias an impressive Franciscan chapel has been built on the Mount of Beatitudes, upon which steep hillside it is considered that Christ preached the immortal Beatitudes.

My children and I often sat with parties of nuns by the lakeside, with Franciscans in their brown habits and those of the Order of Sion in their white robes. I liked their company. Their calm and repose, strikingly combined with power of personality, was always impressive.

Summer in Galilee

The Order of Sion worked especially for the good of the Jews, and a party of them from France, sitting with me by the Lake of Galilee, told me how they had toiled in Paris during the Nazi occupation of France to save Jewish families from the gas chambers.

I told them that my Uncle Raphael and Aunt Louise, of Turkish nationality, had been taken from Paris and had never returned. I can never forget their terrible deaths. I think of them often in moments of my own personal happiness. I think likewise of my young brother Nissim's death on the Island of Crete during the Second World War.

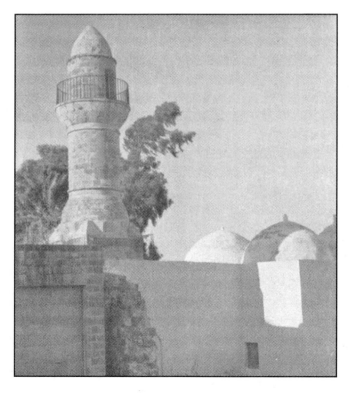

Arab mosque (now Tiberias Museum)

Rafik and Luz liked the company of the nuns. They petted my children and we found them to be people filled with laughter. They helped us to search for old beads and other small antiquities to be found amongst the shingle on the south shore where formerly had stood one of the principal parts of Herod's city.

It was always the visiting nuns whom we met there. The resident ones from the monasteries I only saw in the market, shopping, and they seemed to wilt in their hot voluminous clothes in that torrid climate, as the leafy things wilted on the market stalls.

When Rafik and Luz saw nuns by the lake they would shout out to me: "Nuns! Nuns! Lovely Nuns!" – and run to them of their own accord to try and speak with them in their childish Hebrew. All whom I met, I admired: the fine, often noble faces, the calm eyes, and yet powerful presences. I expect only the chosen ones were able to journey from their often distant lands to the Lake of Galilee, for I have not elsewhere known such fine types of women.

Of missionaries I do not generally approve. Concerning them I shared the opinion of Jan, a Hungarian Jew whom I knew in Tiberias, and who was the father of two young boys, friends of my children. Jan said that as compensation for the sacrifices parents must make for their children, they desire them to follow in the chosen religion of their family. The missionaries in their zeal for their own religion, deliberately try to convert children or adults to another faith and other God. Sadness and bitterness enter the family of the converted. Jan declared that all that he required from his two sons was not wisdom or financial success, but that they should grow up to be strict Jews. Hitler had killed his parents in Budapest because they were good Jews. He wanted his sons to increase the religion for which his parents had died.

I have no religion – except that I am a whole-hearted pacifist and do not recognize the belief that the world was made for man alone, but believe that animals have equal rights and should not be killed by man painfully and fearfully, and eaten as food. Indeed, the exploitation of animals has reached such terrible proportions in the world today, in the ruthless use for food and the unnatural treatment of farm animals, also in unnatural and often fiendish medical experiments and even bomb experiments, that this must all prove intolerable to their Creator who made them in such beauty and variety and gave many of them characters of true nobility, that if the existence of this world and planet does end, one reason will surely be the need and desire of their Creator to rescue the animals from the merciless hands of the majority of the human race of the present century.

Because Tiberias has known such an unusually rich portion of momentous history, and been occupied by very many nations, it is understandable that in its surrounding ruins are many interesting bits and pieces of antiquities to be found by those who have the time and patience to search. My two children and I possessed both. My father had searched much of the world for antiquities, especially jewelry, and so, to seek tirelessly with our eyes and with hands probing into the old places, seemed natural for all three of us.

Before coming to Tiberias, we had sought successfully in the New Forest for the old stones and shards of pre-Roman pottery which were to be found in many parts of the forest area near where we lived for nearly three years. Then, in Tiberias, from the day that we found the first small pieces of the mosaics from King Herod's palace, we became daily and ardent searchers along the shores of the Lake of Galilee.

In an old book about the Galilee and Tiberias district there was given a list of the antiquities once found on the northwest shore of the lake, by the ruins of the old synagogue of Kerateh, buried in a dolman. This read:

Two silver bracelets, one silver ring, two glass beads of Roman or later date, four worked flints and potsherd, one cornelian bead, two silver buttons (Roman), one bronze ring, one faience ring, fragments of faience bracelet, iron nails and light strikers, iron arrow head, bronze ring.

Our list by the time of our last day in Tiberias (for we were seekers up to our last day there) was not as ambitious as the book's list, but was sufficient to have the praise of the keepers of the museum of Tiberias, who purchased two pieces from us. The list was as follows:

- Pieces of Herod mosaics, nearly one hundred
- Seven old bead fragments
- Thirty whole beads (not matching) including one cornelian of large, triangular shape
- Five old Roman glasses of very primitive shape, many stone ones of yellow, green, rose, red, and lime
- One blue faience ring
- Many fragments of faience bracelets, all blue
- Part of an old seal (jade)
- One Stone Age basalt fertility rites stone (female)
- Many old basalt weapons, clubs, axe-heads, tomahawks
- Two large stone urns
- A Bronze Age girl's bracelet
- Two cosmetic dishes of thumb size, for mascara or rouge; one of rose-colored pottery shaded blue
- Numerous fragments of exquisite old Roman and Venetian glass, many treated with copper and other metals
- Many fragments of old pottery in beautiful colors taken from nature: soft greens, yellows, and browns
- Two pieces of red pottery with a peculiar triangular pattern; and one of gray with inlaid design of date palm leaves (these three much praised by the experts)
- One large portion of a seventh-century Arabian pot fitted with a stone stopper of corkscrew form, in place of the later wood or cork stopper, the pot worked with a leaf design in pale yellows and green (purchased from us by Tiberias museum).

- A scent flask, entirely unbroken, of mandolin shape, of the King Herod period.

I shall always remember the finding of that scent flask! There had come a great storm over the lake while we were in our room in the old town. "Run to the lake," I said to my children, as I have said many times when in Tiberias, "there will be things to be found!"

We hurried then to the southern shore to search amongst the Agrippa ruined pillars. Workmen had been digging above there, laying an irrigation pipe along the roadside above. I felt that that was where I must search. I dug the loose surface as always with my fingers, not wanting to risk breaking anything very old. It was not difficult digging that time. At quite shallow depth my fingers touched a round, hard object, and I had found the scent flask.

My eyes told me at once that I had unearthed something precious. Only a few inches in size, it was shaped like a mandolin, with the flask round and the neck long, all of perfect proportions. Upon it was the glaze of great age, that peculiar iridescence, as if it had been painted with shining dust from butterfly wings. When I held the flask to my nostrils I could smell a faint perfume, almost of violets. Other persons who have been shown the flask have also agreed that an aroma of scent yet lingers within; and yet that flask from the time of King Herod was then nearly two thousand years old! Its long burial had protected it from entire loss of scent.

The finding of the scent flask nearly at the end of our time in Tiberias justified the state of my hands, which were an astonishment to my friends in Tiberias. Over a half-year of searching for antiquities there, using my bare hands, had worn finger-nails down to the flesh and stained and roughened the skin over the entire inner sides. I was often asked how a young woman could tolerate having her hands in such an unsightly state! My children's hands were also very roughened, but not as marred as my own.

Before leaving Tiberias I took all our finds to the museum of the town – except the scent flask, our collection of old beads, and my best fragments of glass and pottery, which I wanted to keep and which were lightweight enough to travel with me. I left a message with our collection that the museum could have anything which was of interest to them.

I like the museum of Tiberias; it has the true air of Galilee upon it. It is housed in a wonderful old Arab mosque by the main waterfront, where the green- and blue-painted fishing boats lie in the shade of the pepper trees during the daylight hours – the pepper trees beautiful in the summertime with their masses of crimson blossoms amongst the rich jade leaves.

The mosque has the name of *Misgad* in Hebrew and *Giamic* in Arabic – *Giamic* meaning a place where friends meet. It is a building of many domes, all of the Umayyad, tulip-bulb shape, which, since the time of the conqueror Tamerlane has been a distinguishing feature of Moslem mosque architecture, and is also often used by the Russian Orthodox Church in its sacred building (see photo, page 56).

It was during Tamerlane's world conquest that he saw the dome of the Umayyad mosque of Damascus resting like a tulip bulb over the city and looking, to his weakened eyes of his old age, as if, in its beauty, it was made of the very substance of the white clouds themselves, which seemed its companions high in the Damascus sky. In the museum court there is the rich-scented Palestinian jasmine climbing over old walls, with also a date palm and eucalyptus tree to give dark shade.

The museum is in the hands of an enthusiastic man and his wife. Tirza, the wife, I came to know quite well. The museum is small and not overstocked, but everything to be seen there is admirable. I admired all, from the old map of Galilee hanging on the wall by the museum door, to the portions of mosaics, the stone carvings, the collection of old household ware, the ancient Arabic pottery of those soft nature colors such as I found in fragments amongst the lake shingle, and then, in a special case, three glass vases: small and slender, of perfect proportions and possessing the glaze of extreme age. They were marked as possible third century A.D.

I saw that old glass collection some time before I found my Herod scent flask, and admired it most of everything in the museum; therefore my own find proved very pleasing to me.

From our collection, the museum purchased the fertility rite stone which I had found at the base of a big rock near the north shore of the lake, also Luz's find of the Arabian pottery piece with the stone stopper attached. Tirza was enthusiastic about the pottery and said to me that "it was a stroke of genius to have brought such a perfect thing out of the lake."

I told her that I had not been the finder, but a three-year-old girl! I told her also about Rafik's many old beads and my scent flask, and she arranged for her husband to go with her to our room and see everything. I was pleased to be having such interesting visitors, and felt again that my unsightly hands had not been without their reward.

Luz had brought the big piece of pottery out from the lake on the south shore, after a storm. She had given her usual summoning cry of: "Something very old, Mama."

As she put the old thing down on the pebbles, it was already broken from the lake, and more shards fell away. The pot possessed a fine scratched pattern, giving an impression of palm leaves. Green and yellow dyes seemingly had been rubbed into the design. The neck of the flask, as I have said, was stoppered with a very original piece of spiral-twisting pottery. Over all was that peculiar and alluring glaze of great age. I knew that that find was really rare, and to increase its rareness, I kept only the big perfect piece with the stopper attached, and flung back into the lake the several broken fragments. It was a stupid action, and only the excitement of the find could excuse this. But then I never knew that the piece would be chosen by the museum people, and we would be left without any relic of it for ourselves.

As soon as Tirza had taken the Arab pot, I went to the lake to search for the pieces which I had flung back into the water. I knew the exact place where I had returned them, and I swam slowly to and fro, searching. In the limpid water of the Lake of Galilee it is usually possible to see clearly everything which lies at the bottom. I have often watched young men from Tiberias swimming slowly along within sight of the south shore, searching for the blue stones which are said to exist at the bottom of the lake, and which may be of a lapis lazuli type, and are as big as unshelled almonds. Moise, my friend from Cairo, was one who swam for the blue stones through countless hours. He never found one, nor did I ever see other seekers find any of them.

To and fro I swam, looking for the fragments of the pot, but the lake bottom was empty of all sight of them. I repeated my search through many days without any success, until I understood that the same lake currents which had mysteriously brought the lovely thing to the shore had taken away again the pieces which I had flung back into the Lake.

Later Tirza and her husband came to visit us. They confirmed the age of my scent flask and greatly admired our collection of ancient beads, most of which had been found by Rafik. They agreed that the gray pottery fragment with the inlaid palm-leaf design was one of the best of the things that I was keeping for my own small collection.

I had held a fear that the museum people might claim my scent flask for the museum, when they saw it, despite the fact that it had been found on public rubble and the recent digging of the workmen had brought it so close to the surface that it might well have soon been crushed underfoot by any person treading there. The end of their interesting visit came, and I still held the scent flask. Therefore I decided to give Tirza one of the best of our bead finds, a barrel-shaped bead of rose stone, nearly an inch long. It had been one of my own finds, and I had to avert my eyes as I handed that bead to her.

She accepted it gratefully, exclaiming: "What a beauty it is!" And said then: "How is it possible that you should have found all these beads in a short time, whereas in years I have found very few, and I also have searched."

I replied that I was a botanist and herbalist, therefore with eyes watching the earth during most of my life, and also it was a matter of eccentricity; certainly eccentric to live out by the lake as we had done, through half a year, from near dawn every day to dusk, eating our meals out there; ample time in which to find the old things which the lake threw up occasionally.

Then, a few minutes later, Tirza was telling me a cure for cataract being used by a Bedouin Arab near Tagbha by the north of the lake, where she had her home. She herself has seen successful cures achieved by the Bedouin. I do not think she realized how much I valued being told of that simple cure, the sort of thing for which I seek as I travel. I felt at once that I had been very fully rewarded for giving away the rose stone bead. The cure was simply to apply fresh warm goat dung upon the eyes several times daily until a cure was obtained.

I have cured cataract in the eyes of animals with the use of a brew of the whole plant of greater celandine (*Cheladonium major*), only I felt that the goat dung would be better, for greater celandine works very slowly. [I blend fresh celandine leaves with fresh goat milk, strain, and use as an eye-rinse when treating animals with cataract or corneal scratches. SW] The dung of herbivorous animals has healing and drawing powers. I know English Gypsies who cure lung disorders, including pneumonia, with packs of warm cow dung spread on the chest. I have seen a Gypsy child whose life was saved by that very treatment when a doctor had said that the child could not survive the night. In South Africa, natives heal bad burns with goat dung.

Three days later, Rafik, near one of the old granite pillars of the south shore around which we had searched previously, found the big cornelian bead of which I have written. The lake waves had newly left it there. It surpassed, by far, all the beads in our collection, including the pink one which I had given away! I told my children that I am sure that if I had not given the pink bead we would never have found the wonderful red one. They both agreed that this was likely.

I always enjoyed shopping in the Tiberias street market. In addition to the foodshops along the one main market street, there were also the pavement traders, and they occupied a further place, a court adjoining the main street and quite close to the lake. There the private traders brought their fresh produce from their small-holdings or gardens. These traders sat on the ground with vegetables or fruits piled in front of them. There one could see, in the summer time, mounds of green watermelons and golden sugar melons, smaller mounds of golden or purple figs bedded on their green leaves, green and red heaps of sweet peppers, golden and scarlet pomegranates, pale green maize with stripes of golden where the grain showed through the leafy green layers of its covering and the silken tangle of the tassels. There were smaller heaps of *bamiyeh* (ladies' fingers) — that sweet oriental vegetable with the many seeds held in a natural jelly — of fat, purple eggplants and of marrows. Great gourds covered a large area; and, always at one corner of the market while their season lasted, sat the date-sellers surrounded by a hissing black vapor of flies. Near the date-sellers usually were piled that further food of sweetness, the tall sugar canes: pale green wands with a white inner core of juicy sugar. Then there were also the traders with their wares in baskets, sacks, or big jars; sellers of eggs, sunflower seeds, corn, almonds, olives, or bunched herbs such as parsley, mint, or *altabacca.*

I purchased much from the turbaned Yemenite Jews. They mostly had the look of Gypsies upon them, the typical darkness and the slenderness, and the intense, deep eyes; only the men differed from Gypsies in their long oiled earlocks.

I purchased also much from the Arabs, who were allowed to come into the Tiberias street market to trade. They, like the Yemenites, were often very beautiful and brought sweet shy children with them, wayward as gazelles. Many of the Arab traders were Bedouins from Toobah, and sold excellent pomegranates, figs, and maize. Toobah is a prosperous and large Bedouin Arab village in the hills of northern Galilee, near the old tobacco-growing settlement of Rosh Pinah, and I had known that village and its sheikh, Abou Yussef, in my first visit to Galilee. I always asked the Bedouin traders if they were from Toobah, and when they affirmed this I asked about their sheikh. For their part they seemed to remember me and always gave me very good measure of their produce!

I purchased from the primitive traders before all others, because I like produce cultivated by such methods as contrasted with mass-produced crops grown on tractor-cultivated land, pipe-laid irrigation, and constant use of harsh chemical fertilizers – indeed, all the mess of modern cultivation, which all the world, or most of the world, praises, but which produces food without true type or taste: apples without their apple scent, and fruits which turn bad within a day of marketing, wheat so pappy of stalk that its straw can no longer be used for thatching in our modern time, reed having to be used instead.

Observant farmers who love their earth and preserve its health for the succeeding generations have noticed that the richness and vitality of the soil becomes increasingly diminished with annual application of chemicals, that the rank varieties of weeds increase (especially dock, plantain, and thistle) and the fertility herbs, especially the spring flowers, bulbous or rooted, and the various clovers and vetches, gradually disappear, as likewise do autumn crops of mushrooms of all kinds. Bees and other beneficial insects neglect such land; earthworms diminish in numbers.

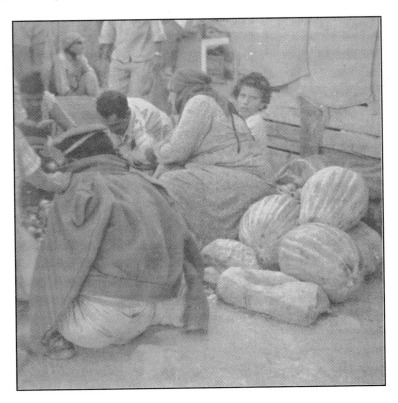

Street market in Tiberias

Now in contrast to the gentle manners and honesty of the Yemenite men, their women were often rapacious and dishonest. They had a habit of asking for the money for their produce before the purchasing began, then delaying a long time over the weighing out or the sorting out of bunched produce, and finally handing out the chosen produce to the purchaser and at the same time asking for payment: indeed demanding to be paid twice! On the client declaring that the money was already paid, there come from the seller shrieks of "Robber! Deceiver!" and so forth. Naturally the purchaser has difficulty in proving that money has been paid.

I had been warned about this and therefore was always careful to receive my purchases from the Yemenite women traders in the market before paying them money. Once I forgot, and I was caught in the trick! It was only for a bunch of mint of value approximately eleven pence in English money. But it was a fine bunch I had selected; I wanted it, and I was determined to have it! My protest to the woman that I had paid brought forth the expected cries of "robber" and "plunderer."

A crowd gathered around seller and purchaser, and all over a bunch of mint! Among them was a finely dressed, good-looking young North African Jewish woman, who told me in quick French to leave the mint for now, but to return in a few minutes as soon as the seller was occupied with someone else. Then I was to snatch my purchase and run. "Take double for the one that you paid," she urged, "it will teach a needed lesson when she counts her mint bunches left to her, and the money earned!" I did exactly that, and we ate much mint for several days.

The only shopping times which I did not enjoy were near the end of summer, when there was a shortage of tomatoes and it was impossible to get close to greengrocer shops; all purchases had to be made from the street-side traders. The big tomato gatherings consisted of furious and excited women in such numbers that all entry to the shops was barred. Although there was much else available in fruits and vegetables, tomatoes were in short supply, and the women of Tiberias wanted tomatoes. When tomatoes came in for sale, the shopkeepers had to erect barricades of boxes to protect themselves from the determined women. We who were in no particular need of tomatoes could not get served with anything else at all. The North African women were blamed and the Kurdistan women were blamed! Personally I saw women from all countries in the tomato fights.

The many wayside food booths of Tiberias were a joy to my children, although we seldom had much money to spend there. But we could look, and we could talk, for we had friends amongst the booth-keepers, many of them being Turks. From such places could be purchased all types of oriental sweetmeats and every kind of nut roasted and salted, popped corn, coated with sugar of many colors, the popular roasted and salted melon pips, sunflower seeds, bars of the delicious sesame seed *halva*, and flat round loaves of bread sprinkled with poppy seeds which could be split down the center to hold chopped fried vegetables of many kinds. There were also curbside sellers of boiled corn on the cob, bringing out the cobs steaming hot from drums of water. I always felt that such hot food was out of place in the summer heat of Tiberias, and that maize is much nicer eaten raw from the fields.

We did, though, much patronize the curbside sellers of cactus fruits. Those "figs of Barbary" are plentiful in Galilee. They grow out from the fat, succulent (*Opuntia*) cactus leaves [also called *nopal* or *sabra* cactus], and are covered with fine hairs which enter human or animal skin and set up much irritation. The fruit is ripe in July, and after being knocked down from the leaves, the "sabras" are rubbed in sand to remove the hairs, then washed free of grit in water, and then, being ready to eat, are cut top and bottom lengthwise, and peeled easily free of the skin. Much trouble! But the delicious taste of the juicy, golden fruit and its cool feel in the mouth make it a favorite with all who know it.

Everyone seemed to buy foods and eat them along the pavement in Tiberias. That custom suited me very well. I have eaten a large proportion of my meals on foot! The chicken market was a big and prosperous concern, as chickens were a very popular food in Tiberias. Poultry was usually purchased alive. After much prodding and pulling to judge for plumpness and tenderness, the selected birds were carried around by their purchasers during further shopping – carried by their tied legs with their heads hanging downwards. Sometimes they were pushed more comfortably into shopping bags with their heads looking out; but that was rare.

I could not bear to meet the bright eyes of the poultry. Sometimes, yet fully alive, they were piled up on the pavement in the hot sun as if a mere lot of melons awaiting sale. Their tied legs prevented escape. The flies gathered on them. Once I met in the market place a Spanish-speaking friend from Greece, carrying a pair of beautiful russet-plumed live cockerels – so big they, and so short of height their purchaser, that the cockerels' heads hit the pavement. I asked my friend how she would like to be carried for a long time by her legs with her head hanging down! She replied: "My dear girl, who thinks about such things? Animals are made for us to eat. These two will soon be in my cooking pot. A few hours of discomfort will soon be forgotten by them then."

She was hurrying for a bus to Kiryat Samuel; therefore I could not delay her to tell her what I know about poultry and their sensitive feelings. But I called after her: "Well, at least make your cockerels more comfortable when you get into the bus. Do turn them up the natural way!"

That trade in live poultry is general in most oriental countries. Chickens are as sensitive and as nervous as other birds and animals. I could write a book entirely about animals and their feelings, as I have known them, only I do not want to be a writer of many books. I write laboriously and have difficulty in finding time. I think that descriptions of animals as a family, their feelings also for a man, have been very well done by Felix Salten in his classic book, *Bambi,* as good reading for adults as for children. We who love animals, who really love them profoundly, are scorned as sentimental. Love for most things in modern times is called sentimental. I think in the present day one is only expected really to love oneself, or perhaps further one's own family also! I shall write here solely about poultry, with a few remarks more on mules and goats which were also very evident in Tiberias life.

When I lived in Mexico I could not keep a dog as I was traveling far. I made friends with all the cows around Professor Edmund Szekely's ranch where I was studying, but I wanted some animal to keep in my house. Professor Szekely is a very sympathetic and wise person, and loves animals. I asked him if I could keep in my one-room adobe dwelling, a hen and her half-dozen chicks which she had recently hatched. He agreed, so Dolores, the hen, and her children of many colors came to share my home. Dolores gave me many a lesson in a mother's wise care of her children and her disciplining of them. For instance, she would not allow them to break the rule common to most birds (except some species of prey) not to eat any food after dusk. Sometimes, forgetful of this rule, I sprinkled maize or wheat into the big basket which was used nightly by the hen and chicks. The chicks would have eaten, but their mother forbade them and they obeyed.

The professor's giant cat went by my house every early morning for his hunting in the mountains. The professor had warned me that his cat was a hunter, and to protect the chicks carefully from him. The cat did not discover for a week that I had the hen and family in my home. One morning he put his savage head around my door. Dolores, calling to her chicks, flew bravely at the big cat. I lifted the hen up on to the safety of my bed, and then spread an old cloth and had all the chicks up also. Dolores requested me to do the same every morning and she knew better than I did the times of the cat's early passing-by, and she would often call me into wakefulness. She was always right; the cat would pass by my door as I was lifting the chicks on to the safety of my bed. That is only part of what I learned from the Mexican hen.

When I discussed the big trade in live poultry in Tiberias with Mr. Ezra Meyer there, who is a lover of animals, he told me the story of a hen which puts man to shame. His story concerned a hen and a boxer dog belonging to a Dr. Isaacs of Haifa, of Mr. Meyer's own family. The hen became lame and lived apart from the other poultry, eventually daring to make her home amongst the straw of the boxer's kennel; the big dog accepted this and began to guard the lame hen and share his food with her.

The hen fattened well on the boxer's food and after several months was killed for eating at the household table. That night the boxer refused the chicken bones and soup usually fed to him with bread. Chicken bones are not good for dogs, but that boxer apparently took no harm from them. Boxers are greedy eaters, and the Haifa one always ate well. It was such an unusual thing for the dog to leave all his meal, that Dr. Isaacs made inquiries, and found that the chicken bones which were refused by the boxer were those of his kennel friend.

It seemed remarkable that the dog should know the bones of his friend firstly, and further should show the sensitivity of refusing to eat something he had loved. Therefore the same food was offered to the dog the next evening and was again rejected, the dog slinking away from his dish and obviously distressed. Other food was then brought to the dog who had been two days without eating; he ate up that food well and did not refuse other chicken bones. He had, then, definitely refused to eat the bones of his friend; he had known her scent and had protested in that way.

Mr. Meyer told me of a pet which he had – a wild white bantam from the jungle – when he had lived in Baghdad. The bantam had been very difficult to tame, but when it had accepted domestic life it proved to have the habits of a clever dog. It hopped up and down the stairs of the house, knew which rooms the family would be occupying at different times of the day and tapped at door or window when it wished to enter. It guarded the family fiercely with a sharp-pecking beak, and could distinguish strangers from regular callers. It also killed dangerous scorpions and small snakes.

As I write this part of my Galilee book I am in Spain and I own a pet hen again: a black, speckled bantam. She came to me by true chance. The entire family of eight, of which she was one chick, and her finely bred white mother, were wiped out by fowl-pest.

I took over the care of that one surviving chick, though it was half-dead then and completely paralyzed in both legs. I fasted it, giving only water, honey and drops of pressed garlic until its fever had abated, then fed her (it was "her" by this time) on raw grains, fruits and greenstuff. Soon she was hopping on one leg, never very far, but strong in life again.

And the charm of her! She knows the sound of my walk and trills at me with a lark-like sweetness. Salvadora, as I have named her, commands two voice tones: a tuneless squawk when alarmed or annoyed, and a sweet trill of greeting or pleasure. At night she goes into a big basket which I roof over with sacking as protection against cats and rats. Every early morning she trills at me from within the basket and then further through the day when I enter the patio. She shows real affection for me and my children, yet hides away from everyone else. Once more I am impressed by the intelligence of hens.

As I come to this hen-bantam's basket every morning and lift her out, feeling her warm from sleeping as any human baby, I wonder again and again how people can confine such sensitive-natured creatures in stifling battery-houses or carry them alive, by the legs with heads hanging down as they go on their journey to the cooking-pot. I used to think about all this, as I did my shopping in the market of Tiberias, and the bright eyes of the suffering chickens met my own.

There were also sometimes tethered sheep or goats by the butchers' shops, waiting to be taken away for slaughter. Invariably they were left in the full burn of the sun, the butchers forgetful or ignorant or not caring that goats are creatures of woodlands and can suffer from painful sunstroke if kept without any shade through many hours. When it was ewes or nanny goats with their young ones tethered outside the butchers' shops, the mothers would deliberately turn their bodies so as to shade their young from the fierce sun. I watched carefully and saw that the sun-shielding was thoughtful and deliberate.

Well, then! Take the lettuce out of the shopping bag and give it to the mother ewe or goat. Tell the butcher to provide some shade. He will mock and do nothing; but at least tell him! Then hurry away – for the sight is too pitiful to endure longer! Oh, those pleading and apprehensive goat and sheep eyes awaiting the butcher's knife! I write about it in my books as one protest!

I think the Jewish people generally treat animals kindly; their great book of the law, the Talmud, contains much wisdom and sympathy concerning the treatment of animals. Where there is unkindness such as I saw with the chickens and the goats and sheep, the root cause was that the animals were being treated as soulless – even lifeless – merchandise.

The pack animals, also, were often treated like senseless motor vehicles. Too often I saw mules tethered out in the midday sun, still harnessed to a heavy cart, while the drivers sat close by in the shade, taking their meal, at their ease. And in Galilee the summer sun at midday is cruel. It lies in the sky directly overhead and sends down swords of fire which touch the earth with such heat that it becomes painful to walk barefoot.

The lash was used over-frequently. Mules certainly are stubborn, but one cannot lash away stubbornness when it is a characteristic of an animal's nature. The stubbornness only increases.

Once, from our window, my children and I watched a brace of mules being used to remove a load of sand. The cart was certainly too heavily loaded and the mules could not pull it. They reared and plunged and snorted, their mouths frothed and sweat covered their bodies; but they only moved backwards not forwards. They were lashed relentlessly and wrathfully by their drivers who, if they had put some of that lashing strength of their arms to the pushing of the cart along with their mules, might have made a little more progress. The mules in the meanwhile had got a newly planted young orange tree between them and were crushing it to pulp on either side. They seemed to appreciate that their destruction of the tree annoyed their drivers, and they pressed against it in sullen determination and could not be moved away. Soon, unable to watch all this any longer, I told Rafik and Luz that I would demonstrate to the mule-drivers what kindness could do for animals, and I would try and move the mules forward myself.

Then I ran down the stairs and across the street to the mules, and told their drivers that I had owned horses of my own and would like to try moving the mules for them. They were quite pleasant and handed over the many reins to me without any argument. I then called to the mules the old mule cry which we had used on the Sierra Nevada mountain of Spain. They both worked their big ears eagerly. Of course they should have moved forward then in meekness and obedience, and the men and my watching children thus have been taught a lesson in kindness! But that was not to be! The two animals suddenly reared, as if by plan, and lifted me from the ground, almost pulling my arms from their sockets as I held on to the reins. I released them quickly, and the mules showed their long teeth at me, mockingly. Only the men did not mock as they rightly could have done. They merely returned to their lashings and their shouting.

"You'll have to lighten that load," I said to them—ungratefully, for they had not laughed at me, and I should have gone away without further interference.

Eventually I was told by others who, attracted by all the noise, had likewise been watching the mule trouble, that the men had had to half-empty the cart of its load. The mules then rushed forward, leaving the tree a mangled thing which would never bear oranges again.

It was from an Israeli mule-driver in Tiberias that I at last learnt a simple method for giving effective protection from flies to horses, mules, and donkeys. The flies plague pack animals in hot climates, for they are frequently tethered for long periods and are unable to get away from the swarming insect pests. That man, Jose, was a greengrocer, though he was purely a melon seller in those summer months that I knew him. I had noticed, often, the great care he took of his mule. It was easily seen also that he was a man well used to mules.

Jose and his two brothers were all Spanish-speaking Jews from Malaga, the two brothers most handsome, equally expert with mules, and helped Jose in the melon trade. One day I saw Jose dipping a cloth into a big drum standing near a garage, and then rubbing the mule all over with that cloth. Because of the man's skill with mules I was at once interested and hastened to ask him what he was doing. He informed me that he was applying crank oil, the stale waste oil drawn off from motor engines and much disliked by all flies, and a killer of their eggs, yet harmless to pack animals. He had learnt it from Spanish Gypsy mule-dealers. I knew that I was learning something valuable and something new to include in my book on herbal and peasant medicine for domestic animals – *Herbal Handbook for Farm and Stable* – already published by Faber and Faber in 1952, but for which I was constantly collecting new treatments as I traveled.

The crank-oil treatment was not herbal, but it was simple and safe, and judging from its results on Jose's mule, effective. Being a waste product it was within reach of the poorest pack-animal owners when living in collecting distance of the oil.

I wrote about the discovery to Professor Szekely, who has mules, and believes in simple treatments for them and all animals, and for humans also. He replied that he had already seen examples of the effectiveness of the treatment, as he had watched it used by Indians in central Mexico where they also sprayed the fronts of their houses with crank oil to keep away flies.

I feel that the treatment can be made more lasting, healthful and effective, by including one or other of the aromatic plant oils disliked by flies, such as eucalyptus or citronella and others more specialized. [Caution: Some animals, especially cats, react strongly and adversely to the use of essential oils on their bodies.] I have since learned, in Andalusia, of the use of wild ditch-mint as a fly repellent.

I had another Israeli friend who was on terms of great sympathy with his mule; this was the Palestine-born Kubi. His mule Schohorra (the dark lady) was one of our lakeside friends. We were always happy when we heard on the south shore of the lake a downfall of stones and earth, and saw Schohorra coming, being led by Kubi. Kubi himself was big and dark, with a heavy moustache, a typical figure of the Palestinian Jew. Schohorra was brought to the lake for bathing on mornings of intense heat.

After Kubi had swum his mule in a deep part of the lake he would sit on the shingle beside us and tell us about his travels with mules. He knew also Lebanon, which faced us across the lake, mysterious with its towering hills and its look of loneliness. He said that on those hills were groves of cedars, pines, and cypress, which were cold as water wells, even in full summer heat, and how also those hills were fanned by cool breezes and therefore never over-hot.

Schohorra had to be watched as Kubi talked with us, for she was apt suddenly to get down upon her back on the shingle and kick up a dust bath, covering us talkers also with dust! The deep kicking of Schohorra at various times, brought to the shore surface for us several fine pot shards and a few pieces of the old Herod mosaic!

If we wished to leave the lake when Kubi returned to his work, he would lift Rafik, Luz, and me on to the high seat of his cart and drive us back the quite long distance to the house where we lived for most of the time that we knew Kubi. We were usually ready, for we enjoyed those drives, borne along by the swift-paced Schohorra. Kubi did a big trade with his oil cart, for the population of Tiberias were fast giving up their former fires of charcoal for oil-burning cooking stoves.

Further, while on this subject, it was a great rabbi who made his seat at Tiberias who spoke apt words concerning mules, and who was also known for his later compassion for animals, as related in the Talmud. He was Rabbi Judah I, surnamed Ha-Kodesh, the most famous rabbi of all, and of such lasting greatness that when the Jewish people to this day speak of "Rabbi" without adding any name, they always mean Rabbi Judah I. The Rabbi said:

> No one should sit down to his own meals until seeing that all the animals dependent upon his care are provided for.

Most mule-drivers are cruel. They beat their poor beasts unmercifully. Most camel-drivers are upright. They travel through deserts and dangerous places, and have time for meditation and thoughts of God.

Concerning Rabbi Judah's feeling for animals the following is told of him, also in the Talmud:

Rabbi Judah, the Prince [the Prince and the Saint are also his popular names] suffered from a painful illness for many years. His sufferings came to him as the result of an accident. How? A calf was being taken to the slaughter-house when it broke away, hid its head under the skirts of Rabbi Judah, and lowed in terror.

'Go,' said he, 'for this purpose wast thou created.'

Thereupon they said in heaven, 'Since he has no pity, let him suffer.'

Through which incident did his sufferings depart?

In this way: One day Rabbi Judah's maidservant was sweeping the house, and, seeing some young weasels lying there, she made to sweep them away.

'Let them be,' said Rabbi Judah to her. 'It is written: "The Lord is good to all, and His tender mercies are upon all creatures. Ps.145:9 " '

Then they said in heaven, 'Since he is compassionate, let mercy be shown to him and let his sufferings cease.'

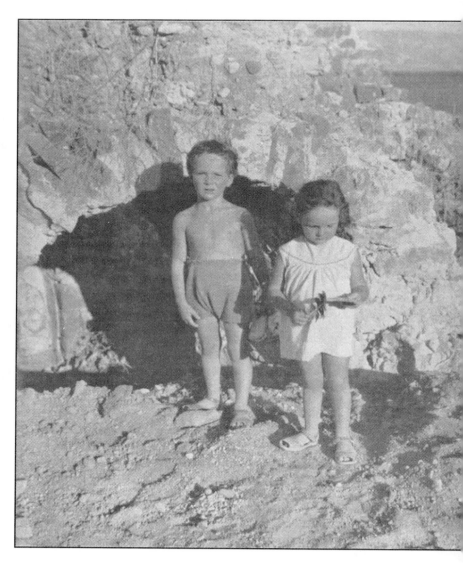

Searching for antiquities: Tiberias

Chapter Four

Festivals in Tiberias

Towards the end of the long summer in Galilee there came many Jewish festivals. The most notable were the Jewish New Year followed by the Fast of Yom Kippur, and then the festival of the booths in the field, Succoth.

Long before the time of the Jewish New Year there were sellers of greeting cards and calendars setting up their stalls along the street sides and selling quantities of both. Artistic ones could be bought in the stationery shops, whereas most of those sold from the street stalls were so tawdry that I wondered how the sellers managed to please their crowding customers.

The only New Year card that I liked enough to buy from the stalls was a small portrait of the Jewish philosopher Maimonides, popularly called Rambam from his initials. We were living then close by his tomb. The greeting card showed the bearded Mogul-looking philosopher, turbaned and gowned in crimson. I liked his fine face and bought many of those picturing him.

Close to the New Year Day itself came the sellers of paper flowers, flags, and fans – fans because the weather yet remained hot, often over 100° F. All those things of flimsy paper were beautiful, being all shades of all colors, and were touched with paints of different hues or with gold or silver.

There were a few lanterns also, in big demand, hanging from lengths of the lake water-canes. I bought a lantern each for my children, a coral-colored one for Rafik and a lilac one for Luz. Each lantern had little windows through which the candle flame in its metal holder shone out like beams from a lighthouse. We carried those lanterns around with us on the New Year Eve, and the big lake moths followed us. So pale they were that we decided those moths looked like the white doves of an enchanted land.

Rich cakes were being sold in the street for New Year happiness and sweetness; they were doused in melted honey and sprinkled with chopped nuts and fruit peels. That was a time to forget the nagging fear of money shortage and to eat several cakes each instead of one solitary one divided among us, which was our usual purchase. There was also a brisk trade in chickens and goats. I averted my eyes from them as always, but Rafik and Luz went to pet them with eager hands and gave the usual plea to me: "Buy one for us to save it from butchers. Buy one! Buy one!"

The New Year goats awaiting slaughter were especially handsome: the pick of the herds. As a goat-lover I could not help but notice some of them and brood upon the vanity of man in destroying such God-made beauty to feed his often uncouth body. Looking about me, I saw no man or woman as lithely built or as noble of head or carriage as any one of those New-Year-selected goats; nor with such beautiful eyes.

The cries of chickens were everywhere, and in the bustle and confusion of the New Year time, some escaped from cages or crates and most of those went tottering along the pavements on weak legs which bent like rubber beneath their plump bodies, for generally they had been reared in the small compartments of the battery houses and had never stood, or run upon the earth, or scratched for insects as nature intended.

In time for the New Year there ripened those delicious fruits, guava, not unlike quince, but possessing soft skins which peel open easily to reveal soft flesh of an almost custard texture when ripe, and colored either cream or pale pink – all very sweet and rich in natural oils and vitamins, and having a scent of such pungency that the very air of Tiberias around the main street was heavy with it.

Guava fruits, tree-fresh dates, white cheese made from the milk of ewes, orange blossom honey, and a loaf of both the round pitah bread, big as the round black hats of the religious Chasidim, and the white bread of the plaited top, sprinkled with the tiny black poppy seeds by bakers for the Sabbath eves and festivals – these were our choice for that New Year feast.

I also bought sugar almonds of attractive colors, including purple, blue, and green, and the sweet honey cakes from the curbside sweetmeats seller. But the price of all food had increased alarmingly for the New Year. Prices were always rising in Tiberias, and there was also always an excuse for the increases. The hot weather had been blamed throughout most of the summer: but were not summers always hot in Tiberias! Then the festivals became the new reason for the elevated prices. A small cabbage was costing approximately the value of three shillings in English money, prunes cost over sixpence each, and the dates that we bought divided out at fourpence each one; a shilling's worth of the white ewe-milk salty cheese was a mere mouthful.

Women with families of similar size to my own alarmed me when they assured me that, using economy, they spent daily on food alone an equivalent of two English pounds. That was impossible for me on a limited travel allowance. I did not want to leave Galilee until I had seen and learnt far more. There were to be many further months there before I would be ready to leave. Watching those rising food prices, I foresaw that the New Year would bring with it hungry days and, therefore, my rejoicing was only half-hearted and flickered like the candle flames in the lanterns my children carried. My fears proved to have reason. Only bread remained cheap and good. A diet of bread with parsley and wild water-mint and dom berries – which grew wild along the lakeside and could be had free merely for the shaking of the tree boughs and the laborious gathering of the small berries – seemed to be a likely diet for us in the future!

"Shanah Tovah! Shanah Tovah!" Happy New Year! Happy New Year! The greeting, always twice given, was called by the people, one to the other, as the New Year came in.

Now the people of Tiberias appeared in their best clothes. The women put flowers in their hair, the heavily scented Damascus roses, prevalent in Tiberias, or sprays of the rich white jasmine, or sprays also of bougainvillea of brilliant shades. Dresses of most of the women were as gaudy as the bougainvillea flowers. The young men came forth wearing bright nylon ties and socks, for display of color matching the women. For contrast there were the quiet black-and-white striped or blue-and-white striped high neck, long tunics of the old men of Tiberias, with their round fez-type hats of black astrakhan [curly wool] or thick-piled velvet. Their trousers were often baggy, old Turkish style, with broad girdles around the waist. They wore Turkish slippers also.

Tiberias has a big population of Arabic-speaking Palestinian Jews, many of ancient lineage: the men tall, handsome, of proud bearing, the women very beautiful, with a Gypsy-like look about their fine features, high of cheek-bones, and with the prominent but delicate nose with wide nostrils. Like oriental Gypsies, they often wear their hair in long plaits over their shoulders, even the old women, and have rich head scarves and an abundance of jewelry. Over-fatness often spoils their appearance, and they sail forth then from their houses like the single billowing-sailed felucca boats. Most of the men speak Hebrew in addition to Arabic; the women, especially the old ones, only Arabic. This old Palestinian Arabic is one of the most musical languages that I have heard, rivaling even that quick Spanish, the Ladino, which the Jews who fled Spain at the time of the Inquisition took with them to many oriental lands – Turkey, Bulgaria, Greece, Rumania, and other countries nearby – and which is now spoken frequently in Israel by the emigrants from those lands.

There remain also in Tiberias families descended from the powerful rabbis who have been nourished in Tiberias ever since Rabbi Ben Yochai removed the ban of uncleanliness and Rabbi Judah transferred the patriate from Jerusalem to Tiberias. Many writers have described these people as seen on Saturdays and festival days, when the men emerge from their hidden homes in the dark alleys of Tiberias, to display their finery: freshly oiled and curled – and often hennaed – ear-locks dangling under their big hats all of fur, or of felt or skin crowns trimmed with fur, fine sables or beaver often being used. They wear caftan gowns of silk or satin, usually of black, but sometimes of midnight blue or tobacco brown, with knickerbockers, and high woolen socks. The Chasidim carry their prayer books and prayer shawls of white-tasseled silk, banded at both ends with light blue or black, within bags richly embroidered by their women.

The festivals were of especial interest in Tiberias, a town always notable for its mixed population, as also is the whole fertile region of Galilee, because on festival days the people were at home and could be seen and observed. Many of them at other times worked far from their homes.

Apart from the Jews from all lands of the world, there were Russians, Italians, Circassians, Armenians, Turkomans, Druze Arabs and other Moslems, and Christians (including Anglo, Greek Orthodox, and Greek Catholic). In Acts 2, the mixed races of Galilee are described:

> Tarthians and Medes, and Elamites, and the dwellers in Mesopotamia, and in Judaea, and Cappadocia and Pontus and Asia, of Phrygia and Pamphylia, of Egypt and the parts of Libya around Cyrene, and

strangers from Rome, Jews and proselytes, Cretans
and Arabs, we all hear them tell in their own languages the wonderful works of God.

Those who possess land in or around Tiberias are mostly
happy, for land in Galilee, with its abundant supplies of sweet
water, has ever been a precious possession to those fortunate enough to hold it. I can well understand the bitterness
of those Arabs who during the Israeli War of Independence,
and then from the following partition, lost their Galilean
homes and land. They will never be able to forget or for-
give, and even if this should come about one day, it will only
be if future generations of the dispossessed are treated fairly.

Of the Jews in Tiberias, apart from the two predomi-
nant types of Old Palestinian and Orthodox Chasidim, I met
with large communities of Ashkenazim and Sephardim. The
former are mostly Jews from central Europe, especially
Germany, Austria, Poland and Russia. In addition to Hebrew they speak an ugly-sounding guttural jargon known as
Yiddish, a German dialect mixed with Hebrew and other
loan words. The latter are known as Sephardic or Spanish-
Portuguese Jews, the name derived from old Hebrew for
Spain, *Sepharad*, and are found in most oriental countries,
and also North Africa.

And then, all around the Lake of Galilee, and in the
surrounding hills, there are settled agricultural colonies of
immigrant Jews from nearly all parts of the world, most of
them connected with the Zionist movement.

Jews of all these kinds were to be seen in Tiberias during
the Jewish New Year festival, which continued for several
days. They came to town to attend the many synagogues of
Tiberias, old and new, also to feast and to hear music. I even
saw black-skinned Jews from remote parts of Africa, and
slit-eyed Jews from China and Japan, also Yemenite Jews,
sightseeing in company with two and three wives to each
man. The Jewish government is trying to end this polygamy

amongst the Yemenites and other oriental Jewish races: an unwise policy many persons think. Several wives to each man is quite general among the Bedouins; but nowadays, owing to high bride-prices, it is usually only the sheikhs who have the maximum of four wives allowed by Islamic law. For my part, being of Turkish origin, polygamy is entirely acceptable to me.

The synagogues were crowded. Nearly all the boys, whether from Ashkenazi or Sephardi families, wore for synagogue a round prayer cap of black satin or velvet, finely embroidered with Jewish symbols such as the Star of David, the seven-branched candlestick, pomegranates, palm leaves, and other Jewish sacred fruits and flowers.

The musicians who came to Tiberias for the New Year festivities and at other times, provided no modern orchestras, either classical or jazz, but small bands of strolling musicians, many of them purely Arab. They would fill the night with their sweet-shrill music and then go onwards elsewhere. Each group usually consisted of a flute player, drummer, and a player of a kind of large violin played with a bow, but held resting on the ground: I was told its name but forget this.

The music they played was heart-stirring; it quickened the sultry purple nights of Tiberias. Once a group of these musicians played by the lake, and I watched them and listened to them through the black fans of date palms, the lake quicksilver with full moonlight to be seen in extreme beauty through the screening palm leaves. Other music heard much during the New Year were the flutes, there being one flute player in nearly every household. Rafik was learning to play quite well in ours. Also many young people played accordions expertly. Only accordion music seemed out of place in Tiberias, perhaps because I always associate this instrument with the rowdy seamen's bars found in Marseilles, where some of the best accordion music and French or Gypsy singing can be enjoyed.

The musicians played in Tiberias the whole New Year night through, and I listened to them most of that time, reveling in such music and only sad that it was to be heard so infrequently. The next festival to be held in Tiberias was the Day of Atonement, following very soon after the New Year. But as that was a time of penance, it was improbable that the players would be heard again then.

The cool of the New Year dusk in Tiberias, when the family flutes were playing, was a time when many a household planted a Shanah Tovah tree. It has long been traditional in Israel to plant birthday trees for the children: a cedar or an almond for a boy, a pine tree or pomegranate for a girl, and these trees are thus considered sexual symbols.

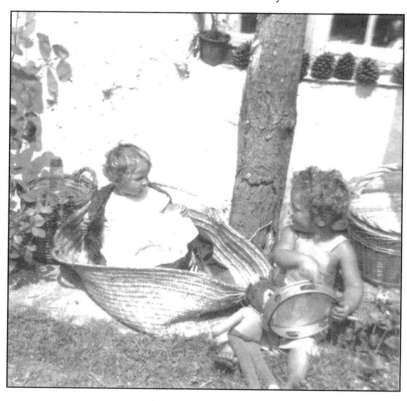

Luz, in basket, and Rafik make music

The Jewish Day of Atonement, or Yom Kippur, is always ten days after the New Year Day, and therefore also at the end of the long summer in Tiberias. That intervening week is a time for universal almsgiving. The poor arrive from everywhere. I always noticed that the beggars in Israel were very generously treated. Jewish charity is famous and sincere. Indeed, as I went by the filled begging plates of the Tiberias poor, with my own purse often almost empty, I envied them many times!

As the tomb of the great and beloved Rabbi Meir — who, above all, spoke for the poor ("If any man will give charity in my name I will plead with God for him," are famous words of his) — is in Tiberias, it was to be expected that in Tiberias the charity would be abundant.

On the eve of Yom Kippur also everyone seemed to be bathing in the lake, a form of ritual bathing, soap being used by many persons. The religious men, the Chasidim, bathed also, their round black hats hung like strange fruits on the tree boughs along the lake shore.

Everyone in Tiberias, previous to the evening feast, was buying watermelons and other fruits. There had been a keen trade in chickens for days before, and close up to the hour of the feast itself. Salty foods and sweet foods were not to be eaten because they provoked thirst. Countless loaves of new bread were being brought into the homes, and quantities of rice prepared for sustenance. The man of the house where we then lived sat down to a meal on the eve of Yom Kippur which, for its size, astonished my children so much that they yet talk about it! A big enamel bowl, the family washing-up bowl indeed, was filled to the brim with a mixture of rice, beans, and a whole chicken. The contents must have weighed three or more kilos, that is about six pounds. A new loaf of bread was placed by it, and a large watermelon. This old man of Tiberias in his black-and-white striped tunic, and wearing his black velvet hat as he sat at table, that evening was going to fill his stomach to last him through the fast and beyond! A good plan in theory, but in reality such overeating must create great discomfort from a distended stomach, and the indigestion which would follow.

I relied on watermelon and breads, also the forbidden sweet food, honey, because it is one of my favorite foods, and I hope it is served in heaven! I say breads, because in addition to the usual shop kind, we had been given a round of *gradok* by a Kurdistan friend. It is a wafer-like bread nearly as big as a cart-wheel, and made on a special type of griddle plate over an open fire. It consists of whole wheat flour, salt, and water. It comes off the griddle crisp, thin, bubbly and delicious to eat. Liking all primitive food, I was always very pleased when we obtained some *gradok*.

Now was the time to visit the tombs of the immortal rabbis of Tiberias: Akiba, Meir, Maimonides – they were all there, and many more. As written, the Meir memorial tomb was above the hot springs, the Maimonides tomb was on a hill slope outside the old town, in company with other rabbis there, and that of Akiba ("the Martyr") was far up the Hill of Almonds beyond Kiryat Samuel, close to the flight of eagles.

It was traditional in Tiberias on the morning of the Day of Atonement to rise at dawn to visit one or more of the chosen tombs. I had already been to them all with my children, but I wished to make a return visit to the Maimonides tomb because of my admiration for him and his writings. I also wanted to photograph his tomb for this book, with the people worshipping there for Yom Kippur.

I went therefore early to the tomb. Even in the clear, cold air of early morning the smell of candle wax was pungent and pricked one's nostrils from the countless candles burning by the plain, whitewashed tomb of "Rambam." All around was the murmur of many voices. It is usual to kiss or touch the holy tombs and ask for a blessing and help in personal needs. I did that. I then prepared my camera for photographs.

I had arrived at the tomb at an interesting time; many rabbis were there. One was of importance and he was splendidly dressed in a long caftan of purple-patterned silk of a peacock feather motif, and wearing a big round hat of chestnut velvet trimmed with glowing sables. I decided to photograph the backs of the rabbis at Maimonides's tomb so as not to offend anyone's feelings. I had my camera ready, when strange waving hands appeared in front of my lens, and it was then impossible to take any photographs. I looked up in surprise at such interference and found there the orthodox boys of the lake, grouped around me, deliberately blocking all view in front of me. I had not noticed them sooner in the crowd of people gathered at the tomb. Politely I asked them to go away. They only crowded closer in front of my camera.

"Go away! You! You! You!" I then said, to remind them of our lake encounters and that we had come to respect each other, and it was now their turn to go far from me again. Their fat, white-faced leader was there, mocking me and menacing my camera with his hands and arms, which he swung around in front of me in a windmill motion.

I felt I would have to leave the tomb and its prayers without taking photos, when my eyes saw my basket in which I had carried my camera to protect it from the sun, powerful even in the early morning. Within my basket was a book which I was reading – *Poesie Arabe*... by Camille Alumly – which my sister Esther had sent to me. The slim volume had a white paper cover with a deckle edge, and looked quite like an official document. Quickly following my thought, I pointed to the book and told the youths that there in my basket was my permission from the Israeli Government to take photographs. Interested, the group went to my basket to see the document. It was a matter of minutes only, but I took a photograph speedily and put away my camera in its case. There had been no time to take more than the one photograph (see page 98).

The orthodox youths surged back towards me, very hostile now. Perhaps the word *Arabe* had added to their annoyance. I have long felt that this hatred of one race of people for another is always unreasonable, when all are brothers at least in the eyes of God, who created humans, and made them of different kinds, as the animals and plants are made differently, each to do special work and be suited to the various parts of the earth. I refuse to take part in such quarrels and have my friends amongst Arabs or Russians (then the most unpopular races with most of the world) whenever I wish. A growing number of men and women are likewise rejecting the delusions of nationality, cult, race, and blind hatred and jealousy against all who differ from themselves.

As it was, the Jewish Maimonides himself had had Arab teachers for most of his life, his father choosing Arab masters from the time of Maimonides's childhood in Cordova onwards, and he had married the sister of one of the Moslem royal secretaries to the Sultan Saladin. There was no time to speak about anything of that to these youths, who appeared to be determined to smash my camera.

The rabbis of importance were leaving the tomb just then, and I hurried into the very thick of them and walked away in their midst. The orthodox youths dared not approach me therefore, and I took my camera away in safety.

I had decided while in Tiberias to keep the Fast of Yom Kippur myself; only my children were not to keep it as they were too young and were always thirsty in the persisting summer heat of Tiberias, even though September was ending. I had kept the Jewish fast throughout my late childhood, and my girlhood, and at other times since, in many synagogues in many lands. The blowing of the ram's horn at the ending of the fast was a thrilling sound to me, and one which I expected to remember after death, if the dead possess any memory and continue to think at all about worldly sounds or sights.

My ancestry is almost purely Jewish and I can count rabbis on both sides. Further, on my mother's mother's side from Tetuan in Spanish Morocco there was the great Rabbi Barchelon, and on my father's mother's side from Smyrna, Turkey, another great rabbi, Abulafia, whose full-length portrait, wearing his long coat of dark green velvet trimmed with ermine, and green velvet turban also ermine-trimmed, we used to admire as children in Manchester where it hung in what was known as "the Turkish room," a small room filled with Turkish possessions wherein, I remember, my father liked much to be.

No one can be sure of one's ancestry. And there I was, always loving best the company of Gypsies and other nomad people, and also liking best to live day and night outdoors. So I claim Gypsy blood and the Gypsies, wherever I meet them, claim me as theirs. My family said an emphatic "No!" to this. Only my father would have agreed, for he himself lived like a wandering Gypsy up to his death as a quite young man.

The day of Yom Kippur is supposed to be spent in the synagogue in repentance of one's sins. But, as I always feel more religious in the open air, I took Rafik and Luz to the ruined synagogue on the south shore of the lake, where it was roofless and open to the sun and the lake breezes. And I promised my boy that he would visit another synagogue in the evening, not a ruined one, to witness there the ending of the fast. His little sister would be too tired by then and could play in the house with companions whom she liked, for she was able to speak sufficient Hebrew by the late summer to enjoy playing with Israeli children. Rafik spoke the best Hebrew of the three of us, and I often used him for my interpreter.

A strange thing happened concerning our choice of synagogue. As Tiberias is a Holy City, and also as there live within it, or in its environs, Jews from almost all lands, many synagogues are to be found there. I was told that there are at least twenty. I doubt if there is any other city with so many places of worship, for also in Tiberias are Christian churches and chapels.

Rafik and I went in search of one synagogue. I did not know then that they were numerous. We passed several, none of which attracted me, and then I came to a fourth one, where I felt at once I would like to end my fast of Yom Kippur. The place was close to the lake, standing a little back from the main waterfront where the fishing boats were drawn up beneath the pepper trees. It was an old-looking, simple place, little more than a long barn-type room with an open court outside for the women, thus strictly segregating them from the men praying within the synagogue itself. I noticed gratefully that there were none of the unsightly modern light-fittings which had been a feature of the other synagogues whose open doors we had passed, and within which we had looked, it being lamplight time by then.

I found the altar attractive in the synagogue of my choice. Over where the scrolls were kept, two stars of David had been painted in black, and between them a pair of out-stretched hands in blue. Then over the entire women's court was a rich, pungent, and very pleasing scent of herbs. The scent came also from the synagogue. This, I found, was from a flower of the *Lamiaceae* [mint] family, with small red-purple flowers, resembling an intensely scented type of marjoram. The perfuming of the atmosphere was created by numerous bunches of the herb being rubbed onto foreheads and hands as a help for the fasting people. The herbs were then dropped on to the floor and trampled underfoot, which increased further the scent.

An old lady offered me some sprays of *habbah*, and I took them gratefully. I was conscious of a painful thirst. The hours in the ruined synagogue by the lake, roofless and open to the full heat of the sun had made me over-thirsty, and it had been unwise to be out in the sun so long when unable to drink water because the Yom Kippur fast forbids any drink.

What soon interested me about the people present in this lakeside synagogue was that I could hear them speaking Ladino Spanish to one another in between their praying in Hebrew. I wondered then: To what synagogue I had come? Questioning the women in the court where I sat with them on the stone bench against a wall, I was told it was the Turkish synagogue of Tiberias! It seemed remarkable that, by chance, I had arrived amongst my father's own people. And this became the more remarkable when I was told later of the twenty synagogues of Tiberias. Many of the women sitting by me were from Smyrna and had known my father's family there, and informed me of this as I spoke with them. The interest of all this made me forget my thirst, which had seemed unbearable on first reaching the synagogue.

After nearly an hour there, the word was being passed round the women's court that the shofar horn was soon to be blown. The fast would then be ended. Soon then came those always thrilling blasts of the ram's horn, strong, powerful, triumphant.

Many people began drinking water from bottles which they had stored outside, near the women's court. I was given as much as I cared to drink. I was also given a large bunch of the fragrant *habbah*, because I had admired it during the synagogue service.

Following Yom Kippur there came the first rainstorms, and with the darkening skies and the tempests of rain came also many funerals. My children and I had grown used to the dramatic lakeside funerals: they were made such public affairs. There were usually the crowding mourners, following on all sides of the stretcher on which lay the dead person, with a black sheet covering the corpse. Behind the

corpse-bearers was the empty coffin, carried by other mourners. The funeral crowd would consist of men, women, and
children, all screaming and wailing. Some families employed
professional keeners to lament their dead. These keeners
were women always, and elderly ones, who seated themselves on the floor of the small court by the entrance to the
cemetery, and there beat their heads and breasts and sides,
and screamed like the jackals whose terrible chorus can be
heard most nights in the hills of Galilee.

Far removed from the solemnity of Yom Kippur and
the lakeside funerals of Tiberias, was the joyful festival of
Succoth, the last festival which we were to see that summer
in Galilee. Succoth was a festival in remembrance of the
Exodus of the children of Israel from Egypt under the lead-
ership of their prophet Moses, in remembrance of the time
when their forefathers had lived in booths, all meals being
taken outdoors. Nearly every Jewish home erected its own
booth, and when gardens or courts were not available for
this, verandas were used.

Decorations were even more elaborate than for the Jewish New Year: Garlands of colored paper were hung across
the booths, and paper suns, moons, and stars also, and all
the fruits of summer. The four holy plants of Succoth were
used everywhere, palm, myrtle, *etrog*/citron – the fragrant
sweet lemon fruits on their leafy sprays – and tall lengths of
water-cane instead of willow. The selling of these holy plants
seemed to be entirely in the hands of the Yemenites or the
religious men, the Chasidim. The Yemenites drove their swift
mule carts into Tiberias laden with their fragrant merchandise of the holy plants. Boughs of date palm were also sold
for decoration and food, with the dates hanging like jewels
from their boughs, and they were of all shades from the
many varieties of date palms which grow around the Lake

of Galilee. The date berries passed from a light gold, through reds and browns to near black.

There were fruited boughs of olives for purchase, of the black or green fruits, lengths of sugarcane taller than their sellers, and wonderful pomegranates seemingly kept back especially for the Succoth festival, for they were big as a baby's head, and the flaming color of the Tiberian sun.

After use in the booths most of the fruits would be given to poor persons or to hospitals as a thanks-offering to God for having brought the children of Israel out of their bondage in Egypt in ancient times, and for the rescue of the thousands from the hands of the slaughterer Hitler in recent years, and from the more recent tyranny of Nasser.

The Succoth booth which pleased me best was made by a Kurdistan family on their veranda, overlooking the marketplace. There on the roofing and walls of their booth – made of water-canes – they had hung in addition to bunches of myrtle and bergamots and the fans of palm, bunches of black and green grapes, clusters of all the citrus fruits including boughs bearing the first tangerines of the newly come autumn, then quinces and apples. They had hung vegetables also, gourds and marrows, eggplants and sweet peppers, red and yellow varieties of tomatoes, and immense carrots bearing their tufts of feathery dark green leaves. There were also lengths of maize, the green cobs split to show their golden grains within, growing amongst the grass-like and rustling herbage. In company with them stood many tall stems of sunflowers, some in late giant golden flower, others bearing the flat discs set with the rich, black, crowding seeds.

Finally, across the booth was hung a long cord carrying sheep bells which made music, as the lake breezes, blowing with strength then at summer's ending, shook the bells. There was additional music from bird wings and notes, as sparrows and pigeons stole from the rich and varied produce.

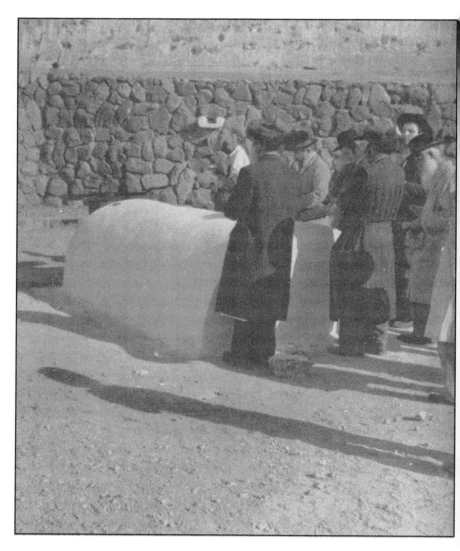

Tomb of Maimonides, Rabbis and Chasidim

Chapter Five

The Rabbis of Tiberias

Tiberias is one of the four holy cities, according to the Jewish Talmud. The three others are Jerusalem, Hebron, and Safed, which means that all of them, excepting Jerusalem, are in Galilee.

This holiness of Tiberias becomes all the more remarkable when it is remembered that that city, as I have described, began its existence under the rabbinical curse of uncleanliness and therefore was a place no religious Jew dared to enter. It became a Roman stronghold, pagan and corrupt, and continued in that way for one and a half centuries. Then, from the time of Rabbi Ben Yochai, it lost its ill repute to soon become a place of holy pilgrimage, and also a place of miracles and legends associated with the famous rabbis who chose to live there: Akiba, Ben Yochai, and Judah.

So far as I could ascertain Maimonides did not have his school there, but he is buried in Tiberias, and therefore will always be associated with the great rabbis of Tiberias. It is uncertain, as I have written, whether Christ ever entered Tiberias, as it remained condemned as unclean during all His years in Galilee. There is a Talmudic belief that when the Messiah of the Jews comes He will arise from the Lake of Galilee at Tiberias, collecting his followers around Him; He will then march to Safed and set up His kingdom there.

In former days groups of Jews used to patrol the shores of the Lake of Galilee waiting for the Messiah's coming.

My children and I never looked for the Messiah when we were by the lake, because I believe that the Messiah has already come and gone, but His teachings and influence remain on earth and will always remain. He took the name of Jesus and then Christ, and was a Galilean Jew.

This is not to be a "religious book." It is a book of personal life in Galilee. Therefore, sufficient to say here that I believe the teachings of Christ are so perfectly suited for the good and happiness of mankind that any nation able to follow them truly would become the greatest on earth, but they are difficult teachings to follow and for that reason no nation, as yet, has ever been a perfect example of Christ's way of life. Christ came to teach the true interpretation of the words of God as given to Moses on Mount Sinai. Terrible things have since been done in the name of Christ, especially the massacres of women and children in the countless pogroms of Europe, the slayers slaying Jews in the name of Christ.

Boris Pasternak, in *Dr. Zhivago*, writing in sympathy with the Jewish people and against the Russian pogroms, laments their rejection of their greatest Jewish prophet:

> This glorious holiday from mediocrity, from the dreary boring constriction of every-day life, was first achieved on their soil, proclaimed in their language, belonged to their race! And they actually saw and heard it and let it go! How could they do it! How could they allow a spirit of such overwhelming power and beauty to go out of them, to leave them, so that when it was enthroned in triumph they were left behind like the empty skin it had cast aside! In whose interest is this voluntary martyrdom? Who stands to gain by keeping it going, so that all these innocent old men and women and children, all these clever kind, humane people should go on being mocked and beaten up throughout the centuries?

I know that the Jewish people believe that to accept Christ as their Messiah means the death of Judaism and their complete dispersal. And yet, since their rejection they have suffered a fateful, diminishing glory. Great material gains have been achieved in Israel, but the spiritual glory – as worded in the Old Testament – has waned.

Many students of religion believe that Christ lived as an Essene – the elect of the people of Israel: a large group of Jewish ascetics, healers, and doctors, known for their great physical endurance and their immunity to pain, able to suffer martyrdom without flinching.

The Essene communities chose to live in the lonely places of the Holy Land, especially by the lakes of the Dead Sea and the Sea of Galilee, and in the hills of Galilee, and further in the desert of the Negev. They lived a chosen primitive life, rising daily at the early time of the Morning Star, to a day of agricultural work, study, and silent communion with the forces of Nature. They bathed daily as a ritual in cold water, wore long white seamless robes such as Christ is known to have worn, and did not cut their hair nor shave. Their diet was completely vegetarian, and they would eat nothing which had been alive, neither flesh nor fish. They never took wine nor strong drink, nor smoked. They often spent their days in fasting, eating only at sunset.

Although the Essenes were a large and influential Jewish sect, it is strange that no mention of them is in the Bible. Therefore, many students of religion consider that the Bible was written by the Essenes themselves. Flavius Josephus mentions the Essenes often in his books concerning the Roman-Jewish wars. Professor Edmond Szekely has written a book about them: *From Enoch to the Dead Sea Scrolls*.

It is interesting and significant that, at a time when humankind was most in need of inspiration and moral beauty, a shepherd should be led miraculously to the cave by the Dead Sea, that great lake linked to the Sea of Galilee by the

River Jordan, and there discover the famous Dead Sea scrolls of the Essenes.

The tomb of Rabbi Akiba can be seen as a white mark high up the Hill of Almonds. His tomb is like that of the other rabbis of Tiberias, with the exception of that of Rabbi Meir, which is in the Sephardi side of the Meir Memorial. These tombs of the great rabbis in Tiberias look like high-roofed, old-fashioned travelers' trunks, and are kept white-washed. Small stones, put there by the pilgrims, are usually piled on them, and there are black smoke stains on the white, from the guttered candles of pilgrims. Such a tomb is Rabbi Akiba's, only it is closer to the sky than that of the other rabbis of Tiberias, up on the Hill of Almonds.

The cave where this Jewish martyr was hiding in the hills of Galilee, and where he met his terrible death of being skinned alive by the Romans, who used iron combs for this operation, can still be found, though it is former Arab guides who know the place best.

It is interesting that in the Holy Land many of the Jewish holy places are sought and visited also by Arab pilgrims who worship there. That is how it should be. The great prophets should be inspiration for the people of all races and religions. It is notable that the Koran of the Moslems praises Christ as a great prophet. The truthfulness of the sites of holy shrines can never be known for sure; some antiquarians declare them to be in one place, others in another. But the adoration of the pilgrims through the centuries has made all those places holy, whether the site be exactly authentic or not.

Rabbi Akiba lived in Galilee during the time of the Roman-Jewish wars. All his life, from childhood up to his fortieth year, he was a shepherd, and all those years he was entirely ignorant of the Jewish Law, of which later he was to become one of the greatest masters. His only fame in his youth was on account of his extraordinary beauty. This beauty gained for the shepherd the passionate love of the daughter of one of the wealthiest landowners in Galilee: Rachel, who became immortal in Jewish history because of the sacrifices she made to enable her husband to study and become a rabbi. As Rachel knew that her people would never allow her to become a shepherd's wife, and that they might harm the shepherd if they discovered her love, she ran away with him and they became wedded – and wedded also to their poverty. Rachel herself was very beautiful and could have married well, but inspired by a great love, she abandoned entirely her former life of security.

One day, years after his marriage to Rachel, Akiba was with his sheep flock in the hills of Galilee, when his attention was held by water dropping from the roof of a cave on to a stone beneath. Where the water had dripped for a long time, a hole had been worn through the stone. This sight gave Akiba a thought which was to alter his life, lead to his martyrdom, and make Jewish history. He reasoned that if water could penetrate a very hard stone through persistent application, likewise could learning penetrate his own head, even though he was far past the normal time for schooling. He longed for learning, and when he discussed with Rachel his idea of acquiring education, he said that he could not bear to die with his mind entirely uneducated. It was decided that he should leave his shepherd work and go away to study. The decision made, Rachel helped her husband throughout and always encouraged him.

The years of Akiba's education were a time of great hardship for man and wife. It is known that Rachel once cut off her plaits of beautiful hair and sold them to buy books for her husband. Towards the end of Akiba's education there was not even a house to shelter Rachel and she lived in a place that she made for herself from water-canes and papyrus grass. Her clothes became so ragged that she was almost naked and only went out by night to find food. Akiba, despite his late entry into education, within a few years had outclassed all other students of the Torah with whom he was studying and, like Jesus, was eventually teaching those who had taught him. His education completed, Akiba returned to thank his wife, from whom he had long been separated.

The former shepherd's great intellect had won deserved acclaim, and the scholar returned home in triumph. But the thin ragged woman, with cropped head, was not allowed to approach near to the great man; the crowding students acclaiming Akiba would not let Rachel reach their master. Only he recognized Rachel, and hastening to her, took her thin hand and told the students that all knowledge which he now possessed he owed to his wife, who had sacrificed everything to make his studies possible. Rachel was then acclaimed with her husband.

Akiba became one of the greatest teachers of the Jews as well as a foremost leader in the Jewish revolt against the Romans. His greatest contribution to Judaism was his unique and brilliant interpretation of the Laws of Moses, which the Jewish people had preserved through their generations by verbal teaching until codified (probably in the third century).

The basis of the Akiba doctrine was that the words of the Torah, in particular those concerned with the Mosaic Laws, possessed a deeper meaning than the accepted one given to them; indeed, that every letter, syllable, and word of the Torah had a more important significance than what was usually taught. Each word possessed an important mystical significance, all of which had to be searched for with meticulous care, and written down. Akiba's own interpretations were so new and fascinating and startling, yet withal impressive, that the Jewish people were in time declaring that the great Akiba saw deeper and with more wisdom than the earlier shepherd Moses, and that the beautiful eyes of this new rabbi must have been blessed indeed by God, that day when, as a shepherd, he beheld the water dropping on to the stone through which it had worn a hole.

Rabbi Akiba furthermore, using his own entirely original method, brought system into the confused material of the Law of Moses, and he was also the first rabbi to codify that great mystical Jewish work — the Mishnah — systematically. This brilliant and original work of Akiba was recognized as of the greatest help to Rabbi Judah I, many years later, who himself became known as the Father of the Mishnah.

The Romans felt that Rabbi Akiba's work with the Mosaic Law would incite the Jewish people to revolt against their Roman rulers; therefore they hated the acclaimed rabbi and watched him with suspicion. Rabbi Akiba is always associated with the Bar Kochba revolt of the Jewish nation against their Roman oppressors (132–155 A.D.). During that time, and for half a century following, the whole of Galilee was a center of Jewish wars against the Romans, as recorded by their chief historian, Flavius Josephus. Akiba and a fellow rabbi, Ben Yochai, led the resistance against the Romans.

The Bar Kochba revolt was named after a brilliant young Jew chosen by Akiba, and of personality almost as fascinating as his own. With such men inspiring the revolt, it was to be expected that the Jewish people rallied to the cause, and they came into Galilee from all parts, by camel caravan and in ships. But all the Jewish patriotism, passion for freedom, and remarkable courage, could not succeed against the army of Romans, who were better trained, better equipped, and ruthless. The Bar Kochba revolt was quelled; the leaders were compelled to hide. They did: in the caves of Galilee. This was the second big revolt of the Jews against the Romans. The first one was punished by ending the existence of Jerusalem as a city for the Jews and the Temple was thereby lost to the nation. The second revolt became occasion and excuse for the Romans to exact far greater penalties.

The name of Judaea was then removed from the maps of the world and Judaea renamed Palestine, being a name derived from the Philistines, the great enemy of the people of Israel throughout their history, to that time. The Jewish nation thereby lost the name of its ancestors.

The Jewish leaders of the revolt were hunted by the bloodhounds of Rome. The search for Rabbi Akiba through the caves of Galilee was ceaseless. It was known that he was continuing to conduct, from his cave hiding place, the lingering stages of the rebellion, above all organizing the escape of the rebels from Roman territory. But he himself would not leave Galilee. When rebels were caught hiding and slain by the sword it was considered merciful, for the Romans subjected the captured Jews to horrible tortures.

After two years of hiding in caves, Akiba was taken. During those years he had become expert in astronomy. The Romans, failing to force Akiba to inform on the other rebels in hiding, including Akiba's chosen leader Bar Kochba, then martyred the great rabbi by skinning him alive, but spared the rabbi's face because the Roman emperor's daughter, having heard of the famous beauty of Akiba, wanted to see his face. It is told that the princess wept bitterly when she saw that most lovely face and protested to the Roman generals that no excuse could justify the killing of a human being so perfect in beauty.

Rabbi Meir, who was to gain fame which approached that of Akiba, whose foremost and favorite disciple he had been, was, in contrast to his master Akiba, a man known for his physical ugliness, though when a man is a performer of miracles, any handicap of physical ugliness is soon forgotten. Rabbi Meir is reported to have performed countless miracles, and his miraculous powers continue into our present time. People were telling me of Rabbi Meir's recent achievements during my latest summer in Galilee.

The troubled times in which he lived and being in Galilee, center of the Roman-Jewish wars, all are favorable to the creation of legends. Rabbi Meir was nearly worshipped, for he was Akiba's chosen successor. He was named Moise, Meir being an honorary name, meaning "enlightened," given to him in praise of his remarkable gifts of scholarship which won for him also the attention and esteem of Akiba. In time his name became Rabbi Meir Ba'al Ha-Nes, the latter meaning miracle-maker. Because of the many miracles attributed to his powers by people who had experienced them, he became known as "the greatest performer of miracles." The rabbi's miracles were acclaimed by the Arabs as much as by the Jews; he came especially to be considered by the Arab fishermen of the Lake of Galilee as their great protector.

He was born in Asia Minor, but spent most of his life in the Holy Land, where, as a great artist in calligraphy, he earned a big income as a copier of Holy Writ. He was the inventor of a new copying ink, which he produced by adding copper vitriol to ordinary ink, giving it greater lasting qualities and causing the writing to sparkle. Then, being in Tiberias, and coming under the influence of the great Rabbi Akiba, he began work on a system of interpreting the Torah which was even deeper and more detailed than that of his master. For many, his work was considered as being too brilliant and involved. However, he gained for himself immortality in Jewish theology with his Mishnah interpretations.

It is told of Rabbi Meir that he died standing up, laughing and singing and declaring that death was the greatest experience that could come to any man, and now he himself was to enjoy this. Where Rabbi Meir stood in death, a great memorial building has been erected in honor of him (see page 111). The building is divided: one leg of Rabbi Meir for the Sephardi Jews, one leg for the Ashkenazi, with separate tombs on each side.

Many Jews are distressed at this division into Ashkenazi and Sephardi, but it does exist, and not only for the tomb of a great rabbi. The Sephardi Jews, mostly of Spanish-Portuguese origin, are recognized as the poets, artists, and philosophers of the Jewish race, and have given to Judaism most of their greatest rabbis, although there are also many gamblers and opportunists amongst the Sephardis, who are often temperamental in their work and lives. Once far in the minority in the new State of Israel, following the big Ashkenazi influx of European Jews resulting from the Hitler persecutions, the Sephardis are now in the majority, and their numbers are rapidly increasing with the teeming peoples of Yemen, North Africa, Iran, Iraq, and Egypt, immigrating to Israel.

It was strange to find my grandfather associated with the tomb of one of the great rabbis of Tiberias, but true. It was my grandfather, Nissim de Bairacli Levy of Smyrna, who built the ornamental marble tomb of Rabbi Meir on the Sephardi side. It is of square form, with a design of fruited olive boughs, lilies, and above all a flower symbolic of Tiberias, the sunflower. I recognized the family touch in the use of flowers; we are flower lovers. I well remember in my childhood outside Manchester in England, the annual making out of the bulb lists to be sent to a firm in Hillegome, Holland – countless tulips, hyacinths, and iris bulbs with poetical names, many cost over a pound each and would be broken down by our big Russian wolfhound chasing after our Irish terrier, often before the blooms reached their full beauty. Then a family crisis would arise: as always, it was threatened that the hound should be sent away on account of the garden! I touched the flowers sculptured on Rabbi Meir's tomb and thought about my grandfather and my father. The words written on the tomb in Hebrew read rather strangely to me. "This monument to Rabbi Meir was donated by the philanthropist Nissim Shlomo Halevy. God bless him. Cithen of Smyrna. God help the people of Smyrna. The year 5682" (1922).

Later, in Paris, my Uncle Maurice, brother to my father, told me the history of my grandfather's building of Rabbi Meir's tomb. My grandfather had a close friend in

Tiberias, a Rabbi El-Hadeff, and visited him frequently in Tiberias. Both men were great admirers of Rabbi Meir, and my grandfather, crying the popular words, "Rabbi Meir, help me!" often had been helped by his power. On a visit in 1921, Rabbi El-Hadeff lamented to my grandfather concerning the state of Rabbi Meir's tomb on the Sephardi side. The roof was broken, and the tomb was being picked to pieces by the hands of the pilgrims who took away fragments as holy relics. My grandfather at that time had come to Tiberias with the intention of buying land there, and had with him money equivalent to nearly three thousand pounds sterling for that purpose. The two friends discussed the idea of using the money to make a new tomb for Rabbi Meir over the old one, and the rest to be put in trust to keep the tomb and help the pilgrims. My grandfather agreed, and as he was an architect and engineer himself, designed and had the tomb built to his own plan. It is a lofty tomb and a beautiful one, and I was content to see my grandfather's name upon it.

I felt that my grandfather's money had been well spent, for any name on that tomb gained immortality for the owner with all the pilgrims kissing the tomb as they came to worship and cry also: "Rabbi Meir, help me! Help us!"

I bought candles from the candle shop below, near the steep steps up to the memorial buildings, one candle for Rabbi Meir, one for my grandfather, whose own burial place is in Paris, and one for an aunt, also in Paris, who had written me to do this for her.

The candle-room behind the tomb was an interesting sight. I have never seen its equal except in the crypt of the Gypsy Saint Sara, beneath the old church of Les Saintes Maries de la Mer in Provence, France. There, at the time of the great Gypsy fiesta in worship of their saint, the small candle-room runs with hot wax and the heat of the place is so intense that it is difficult to enter to offer one's own candles.

The candle-room of the Rabbi Meir tomb also flamed with light and had the heat of a potter's oven. The time when I visited the tomb was approaching the Jewish Holy Week between the New Year and the Fast of Yom Kippur, and pilgrims were crowding to Rabbi Meir.

I have heard about the fervor of Jewish people at the Wailing Wall of Jerusalem. Rabbi Meir's tomb must be the famous wall's near equal. Men and women pressed their bodies over the cold white marble, calling out to the rabbi in strange rapture, kissing the roofs and walls of the tomb, and wailing upon it, and small children followed their parent's example. More and more candles were taken into the candle-room; some of them were of wax, colored light blue or rose, some had a glittering substance embedded into them, making the wax shine as I imagine that stardust would shine. Outside the building, near the altar where sacrifices are made to the rabbi – mostly sheep, goats, and poultry – a thin, pathetic ewe was tethered by the steps, to be sacrificed later.

That morning, while I was there, preparations were being made for a celebration for one more miracle attributed to Rabbi Meir. A middle-aged woman from Tripoli, childless for seventeen years, after offering prayers for a child at the tomb of Rabbi Meir, "the miracle-maker," had borne a son. She was back at the tomb now, with her child grown to three years, and her family with her, to celebrate. According to promises made, she had not cut the hair of the boy until her return to the tomb. That was a typical custom in such cases. The child's hair was now to be cut, and the curls burnt on Rabbi Meir's altar, a feast eaten, and money given to the poor, honoring Rabbi Meir's plea to the Jewish people to protect their poor, and which plea has been heeded well through all the centuries since the rabbi's death.

I saw the long-haired child, solemn-eyed, over-pale, bewildered by all the excitement surrounding him, and molested by the flies which clouded around the family preparing their feast of freshly killed chickens and rice and *bamiyeh* (ladies' fingers).

Many of the pilgrims stayed days or weeks at Rabbi Meir's tomb, praying for his help in personal matters, or merely worshipping him. There are miserable, ramshackle dormitories to house the pilgrims, not nearly accommodations enough to hold a small percentage of them. I was shown, in the library and prayer-room, the plan for new dormitories and a rabbinical school to be built soon on the Rabbi Meir site. The plan was of a magnificent building, oriental in form, with its several tulip-bulb domes in keeping with the

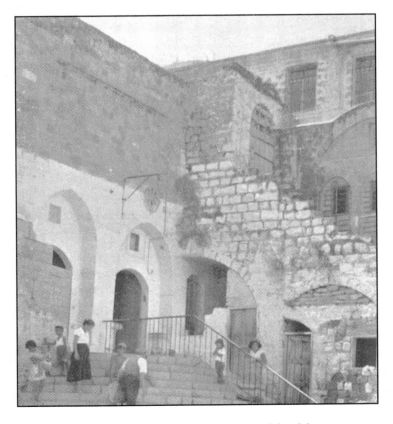

Doorway, Rabbi Meir memorial building

present type of the Rabbi Meir memorial building. I was told also that the money was being given by a Sephardi millionaire now living in New York, who was an admirer of Rabbi Meir, and deplored the hardship suffered by the pilgrims because of the lack of dormitories. He had seen the people, as I saw them, huddled in misery and squalor on the floor by the tomb, molested by the flies. I was pleased that there was to be one new building erected in Israel in keeping with an oriental country. I well remembered the new synagogue in Jerusalem where I attended a sabbath evening service seven years ago; it looked like an amphitheatre for bull-fighting more than for worshipping God.

I spoke to the keeper of Rabbi Meir's tomb. He was a Sephardi Jew of massive girth, supporting his huge stomach on a small table in front of him. He spoke "Spaniolite," the Spanish Ladino dialect, also French, in addition to Hebrew. As he was quite elderly, I asked him if he had known my grandfather. He had known him, and remembered the building of the tomb. He described my grandfather to me accurately; a tall, thin Turk, with blue eyes.

The keeper of the tomb wanted to say prayers for me and my family. Such prayers must be paid for, and my money remained painfully short. Also I am capable of saying my own prayers. These professional praying men are many in all the holy places, and the Hebrew cry for money — *"Kessef! Kessef!"* — comes loud on the ears so that I often thought about Christ chasing the moneychangers from the Temple.

But the Sephardi tomb-keeper was a likeable character and had known my grandfather; therefore I let him pray for me and gave him all that I had, which was approximately seven shillings. Knowing my grandfather's reputation for great wealth I felt that he had expected at least seven pounds from me!

I told him that I was traveling and was short of money. He smiled and patted my head and said that I had eyes like my grandfather, only gray instead of the blue. I told him that I wanted also to see the Ashkenazi side of the Rabbi Meir tomb before leaving the building, and he took me there himself, but said it was not worth looking at.

The Ashkenazi part was downstairs, cool and neat, but certainly uninteresting compared with the Sephardi, splendor alongside squalor, and the passion of the fervent pilgrims crowding there on the other side of the Ashkenazi wall. The tomb was the typical whitewashed traveling-trunk shape. The cry for '*Kessef*' was there also, but I had emptied my purse in the Sephardi building and had nothing for the praying men. One old man prayed for me nevertheless, and I promised myself that when I took my children to Rabbi Meir's tomb before leaving Tiberias, I would give him some payment. I would remember him from his long white beard with the ends of it pushed inside the waistband of his trousers.

Rabbi Meir is also known for his intervention on behalf of the Jewish people at times of national peril. Mme Avigdor told me of one such happening known to her. During the recent Sinai campaign almost all the people of fighting age had left Tiberias to fight the Egyptians. A great army of Arabs was seen beyond Rabbi Meir's memorial building. After a while, the great army turned back, without having attacked Tiberias. Jewish spies heard that the Arabs had retreated because they had seen an army bigger than their own, wearing glittering armor, advancing to meet them from Rabbi Meir's tomb, whereas all that there had been ranged there against them in reality was a group of old men and young boys armed with sticks and stones.

My own experience with Rabbi Meir was when I injured my left leg. I carried a heavy bundle up a steep hill for an old woman: one of those pathetic refugees one meets within Israel, away from her land of birth (it was Greece in her case), bewildered, scorched by the hotter climate of "the Promised Land." At the top of the hill I trod on a fallen piece of date-palm; the sharp end of the branch pierced my leg, entering several inches within. I was lame soon after and the pain became intense. I felt I had ill-deserved the injury, for I had been helping the stranger. I prayed fervently to Rabbi Meir, with the fervor copied from the pilgrims whom I had seen at his tomb: "Rabbi Meir, help me!" I could not be lame! I had my two children to care for, and much work to do. The next morning I hobbled, quite painfully, to the nearest part of the lake where clay was available and plastered my leg with it from ankle to thigh. I continued to pray to Rabbi Meir. I awoke the next morning to find that I had a normal leg. The ugly purple area around the deep flesh puncture had gone, and all the pain along with it.

The tomb of Rabbi Simon Ben Yochai is at Meron, on the hills near Safed in Upper Galilee. Like Rabbi Meir, Ben Yochai has become a legendary figure in Jewish history. Because he had been a leader of importance in the Roman-Jewish war, he, like Rabbi Meir, was forced to spend much of his later life as a fugitive in the caves of Galilee, especially amongst the numerous caves of the Horns of Hattin area, in the historic Pigeons Valley, an area unique in the scenery of Palestine, and which will always be known to the Jews as the Bar Kochba caves because of their association with the second great Jewish rising. From those Bar Kochba caves Ben Yochai directed a part of the rebellion, also taught his many pupils. As a great rabbi, his authority was as powerful as that of Rabbi Akiba, and later, like Rabbi Meir, he was known as a worker of miracles. Every year, to our present time, there is a remarkable annual pilgrimage of the Jewish people to the tomb of Ben Yochai at Meron, made on the day of his death. Torches are carried, great fires lit, flutes and guitars are played. There are many nights of rejoicing. Personal wishes are made as stones are placed upon the rabbi's tomb.

Many sick are carried to the tomb on that night when the rabbi is considered to possess remarkable powers.

Ben Yochai's greatest fame comes from his deed on behalf of the condemned town of Tiberias, unclean for a century and a half. It was sad that a town in so lovely a place by the lake shore should be forbidden to all religious Jews. As already written, the hot springs of Tiberias saved Ben Yochai of an illness diagnosed as fatal, and he in turn put his blessing upon Tiberias and saved it from perpetual degradation. His illness was attributed to his fugitive life in the caves, and when he was restored to health, he honored Tiberias; thus the city – which became the religious center of Jewish life for those who survived the Roman vengeance – was given back to the Jews by one man's moral courage.

Thereafter, Tiberias, on its beautiful site by the lakeside, was chosen by the great Jewish rabbis as the center for study of the Talmud and Mishnah, both, in the manner of Holy Writ, being the lifetime purpose of the many rabbinical schools. Of Tiberias, it is said that the Jewish nation made it one of their holy cities with their tender love from their hearts.

There are two further great rabbis associated with Tiberias, of whom I heard much talk and legend when I was there. Both were visitors to that holy city. The first was Rabbi Judah I, surnamed Ha-Kodesh, and known also as "the Saint" or "the Prince." He transferred his rabbinical school to Tiberias soon after the time of Ben Yochai, and made his patriarch the heart of the reforming Jewish world, and his school the only worthy one for Hebrew religious study. His contributions to the Talmudic knowledge caused him to be considered the greatest rabbi of all, and therefore he is often spoken of merely as "the Rabbi."

He further codified and then perfected the Mishnah, which he built up from the foundations of Rabbis Akiba and

Meir. He possessed a further and different fame being considered as the richest man in all Palestine, so that it was said of Rabbi Judah that the horses in his stables alone were worth more than the treasure in the vaults of the Kings of Persia. Rabbi Judah was as good as he was wealthy, and he gave a worthy example to the Jewish nation in his latter years with his special interest in the welfare of animals: He gave money to youths to buy doves being sold for sacrifice in the synagogues and gave them their freedom.

The other great rabbi was Maimonides, who was brought to Tiberias after his death; his tomb is there. I could not find out whether he was ever in Tiberias. There is every possibility that he was in that city, for he was body physician to Saladin, who conducted most of his campaigns against the Crusaders from Tiberias.

Maimonides, "Rambam," was born in Cordova, Spain, A.D. 1135 and died in Cairo, Egypt, 1204. He instructed that, at the time of his death, his coffin should be put on the back of his favorite camel, and where his camel indicated, there he wished to be buried. Unguided, the camel went along the famous Egypt–Damascus camel road, into Palestine and down to the Lake of Galilee to the town of Tiberias. There, near to the Hill of Almonds and the tomb of Rabbi Akiba, the animal knelt down on a piece of elevated ground. Maimonides was buried in that chosen place, and his tomb brings pilgrims of the world to Tiberias.

Maimonides has the company of many of his foremost disciples buried close by, among them the tomb of one of the earliest great Jewish rabbis: Jochanan Ben Zakai. Moses Ben Maimon is considered the greatest Jewish philosopher, and furthermore, one of the greatest in the history of the world. A popular Jewish saying asserts: "Since Moses there has never been a Moise as wise as Maimonides." He was a multiple genius, for in addition to being a philosopher of extraordinary merit, he was also a great physician – great enough to be appointed as personal physician to the Saracen conqueror Saladin, and later to Saladin's eldest son Sultan Al Afdal. Maimonides was a specialist in the use of herbs, and, like all true herbalists, he used astronomy to employ the herbs to their greatest advantage. He was considered an exceptional astrologer. He was also poet, inventor, and something of a magician. It is said that women sought him like moths the candle flame. It is told of him that, when he was put into prison by the Turks in Egypt, he designed a ship on the wall of his prison and, by the power of the name of his one Jewish God, caused it to be animated, and then flew out of the prison on it. It was perhaps the first idea of an airship!

Maimonides was educated during his childhood by Arabic masters appointed by his father in Cordova. But when Cordova was taken in 1148 by Almohades, a Jew-hater, the position of the Jewish community there was perilous. Maimonides became a wanderer for ten years until he settled in Fez, moving to Cairo five years later, and it was then that his fame grew to its zenith. Soon after his appointment as royal physician to Saladin, he married the sister of Ibn Al Mali, one of the royal secretaries to Saladin. Maimonides always dressed as an Arab, turbaned and wearing the typical tunic, but he never denied his Jewish blood, and in his important philosophical work, *The Guide for the Perplexed*, which strongly influenced his Jewish, Christian and Arab successor philosophers, his aim was to blend biblical rabbinic teaching with world philosophy, especially with that of Aristotle.

Of all the great Jewish figures outside the Bible about whom I read, Maimonides appealed to me the most. My father had likewise admired him, and I had often as a child heard praise of Maimonides. Therefore my children and I went many times to his tomb when we lived close by, for several months, in the Tiberias quarter known as

Maimoneyah: It was like visiting the grave of a friend. We took bunches of the white Palestinian jasmine to his tomb. It is found throughout Andalusia, and also in Cordova, where the Moors introduced it to scent their courts.

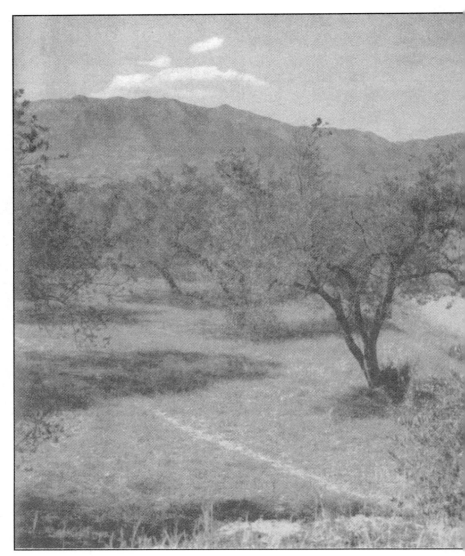

Through the olive groves to the hills

Chapter Six

To Nazareth and Capernaum

Nazareth is a town of the high places. Travelers climbing up from the torrid plains along the Lake of Galilee are refreshed by the cold breezes. The earth is darker there than for miles around the lake, and the vegetation greener. There is an abundance of aromatic herbs covering the rocky ground. Therefore this is a place of goats and sheep, especially goats nowadays and the herds which we saw were predominantly of a black breed, and they passed like raven flocks over the hills, shepherded by white-robed Arabs. There is forestland also, with the great Lord Balfour Memorial Forest planted near Nazareth, to remember that statesman of destiny who kept his promise to the Jews.

The goats and sheep were leaving Nazareth as we approached the town, being taken away to the hill pastures. We were to meet many of them again at midday when they were brought back to rest in the gentler shade given by walls of old churches and mosques, or taken into the many cool stone courts.

The route that the buses take to and from the town of Nazareth is clearly not a natural route to anywhere. The former ancient high roads pass from west to east, one along the foot of the Galilean hills from the south and another through ancient Sepphoris and the Baltang to the north. It is the sanctity of Nazareth which has dragged the road out of its ancient and natural route to mount the steep hills of Nazareth to the holy places which the pilgrims crowd to visit. Only the camels still follow the old ways, and each time that I came to or by Nazareth, I was fortunate to meet camel caravans, sometimes big ones, for I visited during the tobacco-drying season, when the rich tobacco of the hills around Nazareth was being dried in bunches on cords tied between the olive trees, or between low posts more usually, where, as it turned from green to brown, it looked like fishing nets put out to dry.

On my first visit to Nazareth I had my children with me, and there was the usual rejoicing when we met with the camels. The excitement of Rafik and Luz was understandable to me, for I shared their pleasure in the great beasts. Despite their size, they are exceptionally graceful in movement, as swans, though quite ugly when on land, are beautiful when they glide on the water. We met with the camels as we passed through the village of Jaffa of Nazareth. This is one of the most attractive villages in Galilee, with its hedgerows of prickly pear cactus and its interesting inhabitants, especially the women who pass by, many barefoot and wearing the colorful robes peculiar to Nazareth; the younger ones have brilliant-colored dresses, with long, full skirts, floating head scarves, often two and more scarves of different colors being used as a headdress by one person. Many of the older women have a skullcap headdress, low on the brow with a contrasting scarf, often of white or black, draped over, and their long gowns of bright Madonna blues. Royal purple and blue, tangerine and a cyclamen pink were the colors most seen, and how beautiful they looked against the amber flesh of the Arab girls and women, the Arabs now being in the majority in Jaffa of Nazareth and likewise, in Nazareth, replacing the former Greeks and Romans, although many in Nazareth are now Christian Arabs. There were also Druze

Arab women among the others, and they looked almost nun-like in their black gowns and head-scarves of white muslin. Doves flighted above the women passing to and from the fountain with their water pitchers or the more modern petrol cans balanced usually on their heads. There were fawn doves and pied ones, but the most numerous were white as the rain lilies now flowering in abundance over the plains and foothills of Galilee.

At Nazareth we also saw similar crowds of women gathered around the fountain, known as the Fountain of the Virgin, the one water spring of Nazareth.

One of the first memorable scenes that I saw on leaving the Haifa-bound bus from Tiberias, at Nazareth, featured the white doves of the city. On a wall beneath an old white stone house perched a flock of those doves, sunning themselves and fanning out their tails. Above them, against the sill of an old window covered with an iron grill, pressed a pomegranate tree, then in full fruit, each fruit an intense crimson, like fireballs. Above all was the sky of that oriental blue typical of most of the Holy Land, and very sparkling from the cold mountain air of Nazareth. And how cold the air was there, contrasted with the heat of Tiberias, lying its many hundreds of feet below sea level!

It was early morning of late summer when we went to Nazareth, and unprepared for the sudden change of temperature, we had on the thin cotton clothes that we wore always in Tiberias. We shivered in that mountain air and were almost driven to returning to Tiberias without having seen more than the outskirts of Nazareth and that one scene of beauty in doves and pomegranates against white walls. However, we stayed and experienced a day of endless interest. Also the air warmed as the day advanced into golden noon and golden evening.

We went first to Nazareth market to buy a hand-woven water-cane shopping basket, and fruits to put into it; for we had only bread with us. I had been told about the excellence and cheapness of Nazareth fruit. And so it was. I chose guava fruits from a barrow filled with them, only recently wheeled down from the mountains. Cool-fleshed and delicious they were in the eating, and did not have to be well washed to remove fly dirt as is usually necessary in Tiberias market. I chose also big pomegranates, crimson and gold, their sweet juicy seeds bursting through the outer skins, and the leaves, green turning gold, still clustering on their stems.

Zahtar was also bought from a shop where I saw it in a deep barrel. It is a food, or condiment rather, that I love: finely powdered mountain herbs mixed with crushed sesame seeds, to be eaten on bread with olive oil. There is often a certain amount of dried snail shells mixed up with the herbs also, for the white-shelled mountain snails teem upon the aromatic herbs in Galilee, and I had to accept the shells; at least they were empty of the snails! I hoped that they might provide some calcium in the manner of crushed oyster shells, as homeopaths claim.

I bought a big round drum of honey. The seller told us that he was a Christian Arab. He declared: "Who could live in Nazareth with its chiming bells and its power of sacred history, and not become a believer in Christ?" He dipped a piece of wood in drums of honey for us to choose which we liked best. I chose a pale amber honey, with a sugary crust over it. It had the fragrance of bean blossom, and I imagine was made mostly from the nectar of wild vetches, which are numerous in Galilee and much sought by the bees.

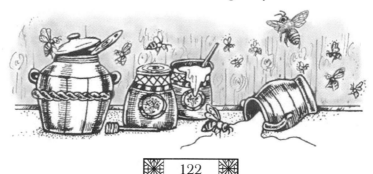

The cold was causing gray clouds, the color of the olive trees, to form in the sky. They were the first clouds that I had seen in months. I was accustomed by then to the always clear skies of Tiberias and its surrounding plains. The influence of the olive trees of Nazareth was everywhere, and not only in the hillocks of its black roots drying outside the small, square houses, together with wood from the bases of the cactus hedges, ready to provide fuel for the coming winter. There were trays of washed olive stones in the souvenir gifts shops, awaiting polishing and threading to make necklaces or rosaries. There were also crucifixes of olive wood, and various ornaments, and even bracelets and earrings; olive wood of Nazareth to be purchased by the hundreds of pilgrims who mount the steep hills to Nazareth. We saw a baby in an olive wood cradle set beneath an olive tree. It is easy to tell the peculiar striped shadings of this wood. The old cradle was beautifully polished and rocked like a small boat as the baby moved. I wondered if the baby would be swaddled in old Jewish and Arab style. My son, after his birth on the island of Djerba in Tunisia, had been kept in swaddling cloths by the old native midwife in charge of me and the child. But I wasted so much time unwinding the long cloths and winding them up again, that I rebelled after three days and kept my baby in a short vest. I was told then, by the people of the island, that the child's legs would surely grow up crooked, as they were deprived of the swaddling.

All around us as we walked the steep, cold cobbled streets of Nazareth, the women passed by like dancers, in flowing clothes and scarves of brilliant colors. They were mostly bringing home water from the Virgin's fountain, for, as in most old oriental countries it was the men who shopped for their households, the women waiting at home with the children — apart from their traditional visits with their pitchers to the fountains or wells, and to do their washing in the troughs nearby, where they would linger in shrill-voiced gossip. We saw so many blue, purple and green gowns and scarves amongst the women, all shades of those three colors, that my children and I agreed that more than dancers, the women of Nazareth resembled the sequined kingfishers of the Lake of Galilee with which we had become very familiar.

There were many beauties among the Nazareth women, young and old. Hebrew and Greek had predominated in the time of Christ; they are replaced, but the beauty remains. Possibly the keen, sweet, mountain air, the good water of the spring, and the exercise of climbing up steep hill roads and paths to the houses, keeps the women's complexions so smooth and honey-colored, and their bodies so graceful.

The men appeared to be of many different types. The tall lean figures in the white or black-and-white striped Arab gowns, with the flowing *keffiyeh* and binding goat's hair *agal*, predominated, but there were also many Jewish types, Christian monks from many churches, and Christian Arabs wearing European-style cloth suits and red fez hats with black tassels. Although their suits were European style, many Arabs, in oriental manner, carried necklaces of beads, especially of ebony or amber, and often tasseled; these they slipped one by one through their fingers when in conversation.

I remember my father also passing beads of amber through his fingers, and after his death in Turkey, I was given his beads, which I still wear; pure, fragrant, and lightweight amber, that alluring substance from the bed of the sea. Along the sands near Acre, a little beyond Galilee, I found at various times, and in all, nearly a half-dozen pieces, of crude amber thrown up by stormy seas. Amber! The Greek myth concerning Phaeton tells that when irate Zeus flung Phaeton in his chariot into the infernal river of Eridan, the sisters of the unfortunate competitor of Zeus were transformed into poplar trees, and for ages shed tears which became amber.

The Arab men of Nazareth seemed to spend many hours at all times of the day, seated at the outdoors tables of the many cafes. The scent of strong coffee was everywhere, and of the sugary mint tea, also much drunk by the Arab people.

There were many bright gardens to be seen in courts or on verandas, these of Spanish style, with carnations, lilies, and geraniums planted in boxes. The geraniums of Nazareth were especially brilliant and notable, doing well in that dry sunlit climate of the temperate mountain breezes.

The first of many places of religious interest that we visited in Nazareth was the building of the Sisters of Nazareth. A modern school has been built alongside where the holy family of Joseph and Mary once lived in an underground dwelling, and where lies Saint Joseph's tomb. Many more sites in Nazareth are claimed to be the former living place of the holy family, and there is no reason why all should not have been. Some families change their homes from time to time, as did my own family, and the holy family seem to have been wanderers, for they had traveled more than most, to and from Egypt, and in many parts of Galilee.

The large, new convent building was square, and solid, as are most of the new buildings in modern lands. But old Palestinian white jasmine beautified the walls as it climbed high to the windows with the glass glittering in the Nazareth sunlight. The convent was a children's school, where the sisters taught religion and general subjects. The voices of children traveled down to us faint as the twitter of young swallows in rooftop nests.

The Mother Superior came to us, stately and impressive, her clothes the fresh white of the surrounding jasmine, and she promised to send a Sister to show us the holy places.

My children and I stood shivering again in the cold air and were thankful indeed when a pleasant-looking round-faced, elderly nun arrived to take us within the old part of the building. Behind her eyeglasses her dark eyes laughed. She seemed filled with good humor, rising up from her as water in fountains. She introduced herself by lifting Rafik and then Luz into her and kissing them warmly, much to their surprise. In such pleasant company we then went to see the old and dark subterranean places where the holy family are believed to have lived, and where lies the tomb of Saint Joseph. All where we visited was strange and impressive, very quiet, dark, and cold, but not so cold as the early morning air on the mountains outside.

We were shown the family living quarters and Saint Joseph the carpenter's workroom. The old water cisterns of the place – now empty of water – were vast, and Saint Joseph's tomb cold and lonely. There was not the feeling of family life as could be sensed in the ruins of King Herod's city which had existed at the same time as the better preserved building in Nazareth which we were then visiting. For among the Herod ruins were the fragments of household vessels and ornaments, whereas in the holy places of Nazareth there was little for the eyes (except in the chapels) other than bare stone. It was difficult to imagine any family living there in so chill and dark a place.

The Sister explained everything to us in an easy mixture of French and English. She took us within Saint Joseph's chapel and knelt in prayer there for a few minutes, and my children knelt at her side.

The crowd of convent children were out in the sunlight of the courtyard when we went back there from out of the darkness of the old places. They thronged around our escort nun, who was obviously a success with all children. Mine said goodbye to her reluctantly; they would have liked her to come farther into Nazareth with us.

This quiet village life of the secluded Nazareth on its healthful hilltop would be an ideal place for rearing children. I saw that those of the convent were ruddy faced and bright eyed. There was the good pure water of the Virgin's Fountain for all to drink. I could understand it having been made a chosen place for the childhood of a Messiah – "He shall be called a Nazarene."

I wanted to see the Church of the Annunciation, especially the Virgin's Column in its setting of oleanders, which had been highly praised to me. On our way there we passed along the chief commercial street, with the small, crowded shops, selling interesting things, handmade wares, woven from papyrus and cane, bales of the brilliant-colored cottons from which the Nazareth women make their anemone-bright clothes. We passed a carpenter's shop and a forge.

The forge kept us there watching by it for quite a while. The blaze of a forge fire is always a fascination, and the clanging music; also we liked the company of the donkeys awaiting shoeing.

Donkeys are numerous in Nazareth, needful for transport up down the steep and slippery streets, and up the hillsides. The donkey is an animal said to be blessed by Christ. There is the form of a dark cross as a marking across the shoulders of many a one of them. There were several donkey colts running at the sides of their dams. Rafik and Luz were allowed to pet them and climb upon them (see page 128). Donkey foals possess long, silky hair, and are irresistible to all children. What child does not love to ride a donkey!

When we finally found our way to the Church of the Annunciation, the first interesting sight was a large area of Byzantine mosaic. Nearby were many new excavations of subterranean dwellings. Excavations have revealed an underground Nazareth, especially around the area where the Virgin Mary is reputed to have lived. These cave-places are beautifully constructed with the original rainwater pipes still intact, and always the big circular water cisterns of tremendous depth; for water has always been one of the first essentials of domestic life for mankind. Of interest was the evidence that since the time of the coming of Christ to Galilee, mankind has known and visited the places of His life and His family's life. All around the site of the Virgin Mary's home are signs of destruction wrought by forces hostile to Christianity, and of rebuilding by the believers. There are many signs of Byzantine interest in this site. And now the Christian Order of the Franciscans are to build a great new church

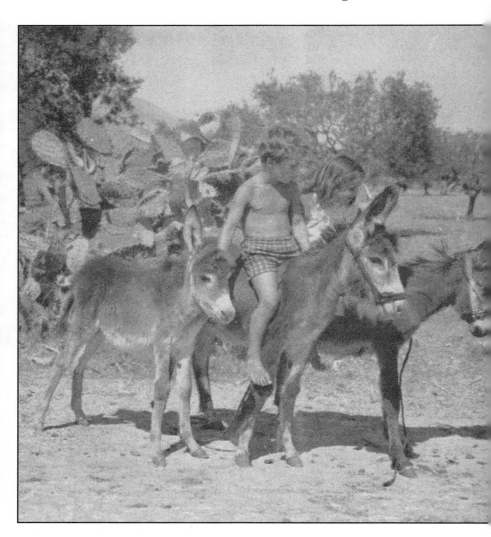

The children (Rafik and Luz) with donkey colts.

over this place. The cornerstone has already been laid. Immense, square and solid it stands there upon a sanctified site. It looks very white as compared with the surrounding old stonework. Everywhere in that area of the Virgin's home was the impression of spaciousness, peace, and survival. It calmed the mind to look upon such places, and I was pleased to have found my way there.

On our way to another Church of Saint Joseph, distant from the small chapel in the convent of the Sisters of Nazareth, we passed the Garden of the Virgin Mary, where the famous Virgin's Column of white stone stands. This is a fine statue, the figure, simple and girlish, clothed in the traditional hooded robe, head slightly bowed, and a hand opened as if to touch the swallows of the late summer day which flighted around the Virgin's Column and land themselves, touching the stone figure with their quick, warm wings. Butterflies also passed through the garden, visiting the fading flowers of summer's ending.

We passed by with delaying feet and looked back many times. We could visit the statue again, but the first look at a place or a fine thing is the one that gives the memory that stays. And we had come at an impressive time; there is a sadness and nostalgia about the ending of every summer of our lives, when one is old enough to give a thought to such matters.

In the big Church of Saint Joseph we were again shown other dwelling rooms of the holy family, who, as I have said, might well have changed their home many times. Here, also, was a carpenter's shop where Joseph worked, and doubtless Jesus had played with the chips of wood as all children like to play around carpenters' shops, and mine did in a friend's shop in Tiberias. Here, again, the home was subterranean; doubtless this dwelling underground had been necessitated by the earth tremors which afflict Nazareth. Such tremors in modern times were cracking many walls of the old church buildings. In Israel I met a memorable personality in a

Carmelite nun, Mary Denise of Christ. She had been one of France's foremost women architects before becoming a Carmelite nun. The Carmelite Order is one of isolation and meditation, a life of the cloisters. But Mary Denise of Christ had been sent to Nazareth to direct repairs of the fissured buildings, especially in the monasteries and other places of religious seclusion.

In a grotto-like place there is an altar and a niche at its side, showing the place where the Archangel Gabriel stood when he appeared to Mary to announce that she was to be the mother of Christ. I will long remember the dove above the altar. I regretted the fixing of electric lights to spoil the dim beauty there.

We stayed in Nazareth until the evening. I took no photographs; it is not possible to photograph "atmosphere." I felt it to be easier to write about Nazareth. But I would like to return one day with paint and many canvases, when I have learned to paint better. As we went away in the always hastening motor-bus, I considered that just as Lourdes has its miracles, the town of Nazareth surely can claim one great miracle: having resisted change. In a noisy modern, rapidly developing new state, Nazareth remains in quiet isolation on its hilltop, with its old places the same as when the holy family lived there, and its life closely the same, with the goat and sheep herds going from and to pastures, the donkeys carrying riders or produce along the steep streets, the camels arriving and leaving, and the doves flighting over house walls and roof-tops. The women still walk with a grace of older times, carrying water-pitchers to and from Nazareth's one fountain; and their children sleep in olive wood rocking cradles, and are rocked by the breezes of the mountains of Galilee. The language of its inhabitants is different – mainly Arabic now, but Hebrew is being spoken there again.

Sometimes, returning late from Haifa, going onwards to Tiberias, I passed by Nazareth in the full moonlight: All the buildings then looked unearthly white in the moonbeams raying over the dark hillside, over which the town is stretched. I think the sacred town appeared more impressive then than at any other time, and exactly as I had imagined since I had first learnt about Nazareth and its history. I always strained my eyes back to see Nazareth as long as I could achieve sight.

It was also late summer when we went to Capernaum. There the purpose was to visit the ancient and famous ruins of the old synagogue, on the northern side of the Lake of Galilee, which was said to have been Christ's favorite part of Galilee, beyond Tagbha and Magdalena. There Christ had lived and preached:

"And leaving Nazareth he came and dwelt in Capernaum, which is upon the coast of the Sea of Galilee on the border of Zebulon and Naphtali." And then:

O land of Zebulon and land of Naphtali, by
the road to the sea, beyond the Jordan, Galilee
of the Gentiles.
The people who sat in darkness have seen a
great light. (Matt. 4:12-16)

Our journey to Capernaum from Tiberias necessitated a half-hour bus journey along the north shore of the lake and through the small village of Migdal, where Mary Magdalene once lived. Then after leaving the bus, a walk of an hour awaited us.

The day proved to be one of exceptional heat; very unlike the one which we had spent at Nazareth only a short time earlier. The road from beyond Migdal to Capernaum goes within sight of the Lake of Galilee for most of the way, but is too far from the lake to be refreshed by its cool breezes. And it is an open road with no shade at all apart from small areas around the dom trees. We rested by each one as we came there, and also we ate quantities of the dom fruits which lay thick upon the thorny branches and were also piled around the roots. The fruits were of such excellent quality that I promised my children that on our return from Capernaum we would stay a while to collect fruits for our forthcoming journey by sea from Haifa to Marseilles.

We passed by an unattractive modern church, where – a notice on the gate informed us – the miracle of "the Five Loaves and Two Fishes" had occurred.

> From whence can a man satisfy these men with bread here in the wilderness? They that had eaten were about four thousand. (Mark 8:4)

Wilderness was all around us, and our eyes therefore kept grateful company with the Franciscan church built high on the hill considered to be the place of the Beatitudes which is known, therefore, as the Mount of the Beatitudes. This Franciscan church is recently built. The octagonal shape is very attractive, and the herb garden surrounding the church is in keeping with the building. The road all the way to Capernaum was deserted, it being too hot a time of the year to attract tourists to the Lake of Galilee.

We saw farther during part of the walk one of the long-deserted forts of the Crusaders, high up on the skyline, making a pathetic, unintended monument to the thousands of Knights of the Cross who were slain by the army of Saladin upon the surrounding hills and plains of this area.

Whenever the road approached close to the lake we were greatly tempted to descend the rough, boulder-strewn land to its shores, and there bathe again in the water which shimmered and lured. But I was sensing that this was snake land, and therefore our bathing must be delayed. The sun continued to blaze like the fire in the blacksmith's forge we were remembering from Nazareth.

Farther on, we came in sight of a far-stretching grove of eucalyptus trees, where I was sure must be Capernaum. The trees at that distance looked very black against the sun-possessed sky.

At the same time we came upon cultivated land close by the lake. A group of men were tilling the earth using horses, making ready for the winter planting as soon as the weather had cooled a little. There were stretches of sweet peppers and tomatoes bearing fruits. Water gushed out from big irrigation pipes. Rafik, Luz and I hastened to those pipes like travelers who had crossed a great desert! We let the water spurt over our dusty faces and limbs. It came warm from the pipes, but pleasant.

The workers were Israelis and Druze Arabs, and as we lingered around the irrigation pipes they came to speak to us. They confirmed that the eucalyptus grove was Capernaum and that it was very cool there. "A breeze-blest place," said one of the workers in English. He was from New Zealand and had lived in Israel three years.

Of the workers who came to speak with us – wondering what we were doing out there, "far from anywhere in the midday sun" – there were one each from Yugoslavia, Sweden, India, and America, one Israeli-born and three Druze Arabs. On my questioning, they told me that they were very happy in Israel despite long working hours on land "possessed by thistles." The Druze Arabs said that conditions were good for their people in Israel.

Only the Indian was dissatisfied. He was from Bombay and had married an English-born girl whom he had met in Israel. They had three children. But he and his wife were miserable on account of the high prices of food and clothing, making it nearly impossible to rear their children properly outside a kibbutz, and his wife would not enter one as she disliked communal life. Therefore, he was trying to save enough from his wages for the fares to take his entire family to India, but it was proving nearly impossible to save anything.

I sympathized with the Jew from India because I know the pain in the heart when one has a driving urge to get to any place but not sufficient money to achieve the journey. Only I told him that I found Galilee, and especially the lands of the lake, very beautiful, and wanted to return there many times. He agreed about the beauty, but deplored again the high prices.

I asked the men about snakes, and they confirmed that they were numerous in that boulder-strewn, thorny area, and cautioned us not to stray far from the road until we reached Capernaum.

Finally, we were told that if we had not yet had our midday meal we could help ourselves to all the peppers, tomatoes, and cucumbers that we wished to eat. We had not yet eaten and therefore accepted the invitation gratefully.

We then went onwards to Capernaum. Only we took care, as we passed more dom trees and ate more fruit from them, to beat around us first for snakes. Snakes like dom trees. They have their holes amongst the spreading roots and prey on the birds and rodents which come to the dom feast which every tree piles in profusion upon the ground. The only big snake that my children and I saw by the Lake of Galilee was driven out of its hole at the foot of a dom tree on the north shore. Boys saw it and dug for it with sticks, having also armed themselves with big stones. Soon a large snake of about four feet in length rushed from its hole in fury as well as fear. Its clever writhings as it moved caused it to escape the flung stones and it speeded towards the lake untouched.

We saw no snakes on our way to Capernaum, and when we at last reached our destination we forgot all about them.

Capernaum! The glory of the place! Out from the noon-day fire of the sun we went, into the cool of the eucalyptus grove with its rustling musical leaves, the near lake showing like tall blue-painted windows in places through the screening gray of eucalyptus.

We stepped as gratefully from the hot road into that area of tree shade, lake airs, and old stone as Christ must have done so many times, thousands of years ago, and likewise the other great rabbis who visited the place – perhaps Akiba, Ben Yochai, Meir, Judah "the Prince," even Maimonides – all of the Great Ones after Christ associated with Galilee. It is said of Capernaum that it was the most important synagogue in all Galilee, and one of the most chosen of ancient Judaea. The ruins of the old synagogue itself are now often called Tel Hum.

We found Franciscans in charge of the place; two of them were reading a sundial in their quiet herb-planted garden as I approached with my children. They opened a locked door to give us entry into the ruins. It is known that Capernaum was once more than a synagogue. It was possibly a lakeside city; certainly it had been a sociable village, and an important religious center. It was the scene of many of Christ's most important miracles and sermons, and He spent much of His adult life there. It is also known to be the native place of at least three of His apostles. The utter destruction of the area is attributed to the severe earthquakes which have visited Galilee frequently, and are, to this day, destroying old buildings or damaging them: hence the visit to Nazareth, as I have told, of architectural experts such as Mary Denise of Christ and others. There are black volcanic boulders scattered close to the site of Capernaum.

We were the sole visitors to the ruins of Capernaum on that day of intense heat; the gates were locked behind us and we were alone there. "Mystery of mysteries," were the words which came to my mind as I looked around me! The position of the ruins showed that the synagogue had once faced the lake, and from its roof and terraces it must have given a wonderful view of a great expanse of the lake and its shores. Like most orthodox synagogues there was evidence of a special court for the women; Jewish women, except in the modern Conservative and Reform synagogues of some western countries, are not allowed within the synagogue, but must view the ceremonies from a court outside, or a balcony above, so they are completely segregated from the menfolk.

When we climbed onto the highest points of the synagogue to look across to the lake, the brilliant sky had clouded over, and there were pale sulfur sunbeams slanting across the misty gray sky down into the lake, which was then dappled with silver light. Green-gray eucalyptus trees and dark pines stretched away to the shimmering waters.

There was a sadness in remembering that that once great synagogue in its exquisite setting had been the chosen one for large gatherings of the ultra-orthodox Pharisees and Scribes who concentrated their attention on opposing all the new and inspired teachings of Christ, every one of which, if truthfully followed, could only have benefited mankind, bringing peace to the world. It was the Synagogue of Capernaum which Jesus described, with cynicism, as "exalted unto heaven."

It has been said of Capernaum that the magnificent synagogue was built by the Roman General Titus for the beautiful Jewish woman, Berenice, whom he loved. That accounts for its unusual richness and lavishness, unlike anything seen in other synagogues: possibly all to please the eyes of a woman. Also there is found in Capernaum, graven on walls and pillars, things not found in any other Jewish synagogue, notably two Roman eagles.

Firstly to be seen graven on the stones of Capernaum are the seven permitted Jewish symbols for holy places – the star of David, the olive branch, the pomegranate fruit, the vine cluster, the menorah (seven-branched candlestick), the eastern star of Solomon, and the lion of Judah. I saw also on the fragments of pillars and different stone parts of the ruins: figs, lemons, apples, pears, date palms with their fruit clusters, the acanthus and the rose, also animal forms other than the lion of Judah, notably the serpent and gazelle, also more birds, doves, and a type of falcon.

If there is any fact in this account of Titus and Berenice, it seems the Jewish Berenice must have told Titus what was permitted in a synagogue, and the Roman Titus then added things of his own ideas, including the eagles. Further, it could be claimed that the total destruction of the synagogue, the reduction of the place to ruins, was the vengeance of Titus when Berenice ceased to love him.

Whilst I was peering around the ruins, searching out the graven symbols, and hoping also that I might find an old bead or a good fragment of old glass or pot, my children were playing at stepping-stones: from ruined piece to ruined piece. I expect it was irreverent, but there was no one there to see them and it was not as if they were playing upon tombs.

Later, Rafik and Luz and I searched rubble heaps behind the synagogue; here there was some evidence of former domestic life in the fragments of old crockery and glass, though none of it was attractive. I found eventually, within one heap, a bead of dark red stone, of size no bigger than an apple seed. Rafik found a shard of fawn-colored pottery with pale blue painting on top, only a fragment, and without value, but a relic of Capernaum worth keeping for its beauty.

All the time, whenever I looked to the left of Tel Hum, I enjoyed the magnificence of the red dome of a Greek Orthodox church, of Moslem mosque shape, similar to the beautiful Greek church in Nazareth. When we left the ruins of Capernaum to return home, I asked the Franciscans about the Greek church. They told me that it had been empty for many years, and that the cattle and sheep were now sheltered in it. Loving cattle and sheep as I do, it did not seem to me to be an ill use for an empty church.

As I walked away from Capernaum, through the late noon beauty of Galilee, I could understand why it was Nature that had provided Jesus with numerous illustrations for His teachings. The climate of Galilee was more suited than any other to itinerant work and open-air preaching. Days of unbroken sunshine and nights of pleasant warmth are usual for seven to eight months of every year, and it is possible, without interference from rain, to gather crowds on those hillsides and plains for most of the year. And the brilliant moonlight of Galilee is a further boon to open-air ministry. I could see the phantom crowds on those hillsides, listening to the powerful words of Galilee's most famous preacher, whose voice has been described as deep and low, and as musical as the waters of Galilee.

The walk to Capernaum had not tired me, and I planned on our return way to Tiberias to climb as close as possible to the Crusader fort which I had seen that morning. Rafik and Luz could be left gathering dom fruits after I had searched first for snakes: for the snakes, if not already there, would not come in the daytime with two chattering children present.

I felt that the site of the Crusader fort had been inspired by Capernaum close by; the Crusaders who had come to Palestine to take their holy Christian places from the infidels wanted to watch over the historic and sacred ruins.

There are many Crusader forts left in the Holy Land. Always poised on high places, in the way of eagle nests, and in the customary way of European forts, scant thought seemed to have been given to escape from the fire of the daily sun or to the vital provision of good water: symbolic, I felt, of the hopeless campaign of an army who did not understand the nature of the land which it had hoped to save. Their medieval iron armor, in which they had clothed themselves for warring beneath such a sun, had been their final folly. The Knights of the Cross had sworn on holy relics to die fighting, and they had largely kept their vows. Thus there died in the field, especially on the plains of Galilee, many of the great princes and dukes, and the heirs of great families from most countries of Europe.

It was in the Horns of Hattin area, between Tiberias and Nazareth, and not far from Capernaum, that in a terrible massacre, one of the cruelest in human history, the Saracens destroyed for all time the power of the Crusaders. Two thousand knights and fifty thousand men on foot were slain; the brushwood of the plains on which the Crusaders fought was set on fire by the Saracens, and the knights roasted alive in their heavy armor. Those who escaped were driven into the Lake of Galilee and drowned, their heavy armor making it impossible to swim.

I thought of all that history as I climbed upwards over the thorny and rocky hill surface towards the fort. I had recently finished, in Tiberias, my reading of the classic *Memoir of the Crusades*. I thought also of those strange characters known as Prester John, the King of Abyssinia, and "The Old Man of the Mountains," who had been given much mention in the *Memoir*. Then of Richard Cœur-de-Lion, who did such mighty deeds in the Crusader wars, and earned such respect from the Saracens that long after, when Saracen or Bedouin horses shied at a bush or tree, their riders would say: "Wisht now. Do you fear that that is King Richard?"

Then I imagined that principal leader in the Crusades, King Louis of France, and how he had been described in the crusades book, serving as justice to his people in his Paris garden, clothed then in a tunic of camlet, with tartan sleeveless surcoat and a mantle of black taffeta about his neck, his hair well combed, and a hat of white peacock feathers upon his head – and who, during the Crusades, had to have the seat of his trousers cut open, as I described earlier, because of the dysentery prevailing amongst the Crusaders. There had been a further terrible sickness afflicting the knights, a type of scurvy due to shortage of fresh fruits and vegetables, essential foods in that climate of the Holy Land.

> The sickness increased amongst the host in a sort that dead flesh was caused to form upon the gums of the mouth, and it became impossible for the host to swallow their food or masticate it, and the barber surgeon had to cut away the dead flesh that formed, and the cry throughout the camp of the people being operated upon sounded more bitter than women laboring of child.

Such things men can endure for a cause in which they believe. Those were strange thoughts as I clambered up the Galilean hillside towards the Crusader fort, but I was accompanied by the thirsty biting flies of the Galil, the flat, silent kind, with the yellow, black-barred wings, and I had no herbs with me to protect my flesh against them. At least the medieval armor of the knights had kept away the biting flies, I told myself!

I approached close enough to the old fort to hear the harsh crying of ravens around it. The sun was setting then, and I dared not leave my children longer alone. I had had sight of them below me all the time of my climb. From the place on the hillside that I had finally reached they had become reduced to a size a little larger than a pair of pigeons.

When I returned to Rafik and Luz they were still gathering dom fruits with busy hands, and they told me about real pigeons which had visited them while I was up the hill. A big flock of wild pigeons had descended upon the dom tree by which I had told them to await my return, and caused a golden rain of dom fruits to fall upon the ground all around the tree. The birds had eaten a few themselves, and then flown away, and left the rest as a gift for the children to eat and gather.

Chapter Seven

A House in Galilee

Seven years ago – before my children were born – I had another summer in Galilee. I lived then in the mountains of the Upper Galil, to the north, and I worked on three different Israeli collective farms or kibbutzim. My work was entirely in the fields, mostly helping to harvest the various summer-time crops; only in the third kibbutz did I work as a shepherd.

The second of those kibbutzim took me near to the old tobacco-growing settlement of Rosh Pinah. There I was also close to the interesting town of Safed, the highest in Galilee, and one of the oldest. Safed was the center of the mysterious Jewish Kabbalists in the sixteenth and seventeenth centuries, and therefore the birthplace of Hebrew mysticism, and seems to have retained a strange brooding atmosphere.

I further had as my nearest village the big Bedouin Arab settlement of Toobah, under the rule of the remarkable and powerful sheikh, Abou Yussef.

Then, for yet more interest, there was the River Jordan and its valley, the river close enough for the sound of its swift waters to be heard faintly or loudly often in the still Galilean nights.

My field-task in the Rosh Pinah kibbutz was the melon harvest, although sometimes there was work with other vegetable crops, notably with a big harvest of onions and garlic.

The kibbutz was short of helpers, especially people for the land, and I liked the place and the work, and wanted to stay there for several months. The one problem for me was that I was without any suitable place in which to sleep, where I could have my big Afghan hound, Fuego, with me, who at that time traveled everywhere at my side. For my first week

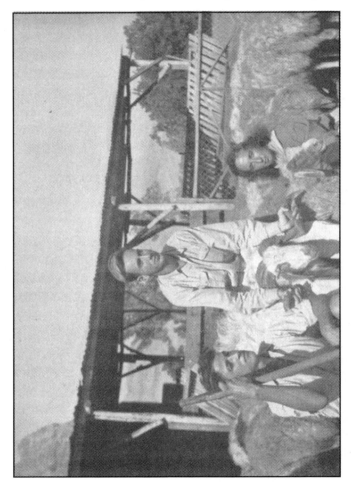

Shepherds of the Turkish kibbutz in Upper Galilee; Juliette on the right

I had been given a tent as a house, a small one for my own use, and in which I could also keep my dog. That had been very pleasing, though it had taken all of my free time for most of the week to clean out the tent of collected debris, dig out the evil-smelling floor, and replace it with fresh earth which had to be beaten flat with a heavy boulder with much toil. I had then collected mountain herbs for strewing on the floor — fennel, sage, and rosemary — and was rejoicing in my possession of a most pleasant dwelling-place, when the former occupants passed by, saw how nice a tent could be made to look, and decided that they would like to return! They were permanent members of the kibbutz, and I was only a traveling worker. Protest against an injustice was useless. I said little but thought much! I did not want to leave the kibbutz, for on the facing hill was an interesting Bedouin village. I longed to visit there, and knew that I would visit as soon as I had learnt some elementary Arabic.

I was offered accommodation in one of the typical kibbutz wooden buildings of that time, where many people shared small cupboard-like rooms made airless by fine wire mosquito guard mesh nailed over all windows. I was told that my hound must be tied up outside. I could not leave my dog tethered alone anywhere in the night, liable to attack from jackals. Nor could I sleep where there was lack of air. Therefore, for a number of nights I lay out on the ground near some rocks for shelter, alongside my dog. Then the ants found us, and by the third night the pricking stings of swarming ants made sleep impossible; we went for a moonlight walk instead, and, as always since I had come to that part of Galilee, I was enchanted by my surroundings.

It was that night that the idea came to me to make habitable one of the deserted and partly wrecked Arab houses abandoned during the recent Jewish War of Independence. There was a long row of those houses on a craggy part of the hillside, overlooking the Jordan Valley. They were a half-hour walk away from the main kibbutz buildings, but the horses were kept in a compound nearby, and also the cattle building was near; some kibbutz workers lived in that vicinity in the usual wooden huts, and therefore I would not be in complete isolation if I went there.

The kibbutz doctor, from Leeds, was friendly towards me and my plan, and said that if I could find a house not too badly ruined he would give me his support to occupy it, provided I could make such a place habitable. Therefore I obtained a day's freedom from work and, accompanied by my dog Fuego, commenced my search. And it was an exciting search.

The Arab houses had been deserted for two years, during which time they had become almost blocked with debris from the falling stones of their tottering walls and plaster from the inner walls also. I knew that bats dwelt there, for I had seen them flitting in the night, from and to those roofless places. Every dwelling that I looked into, my eyes warned me "No" – yet I much wanted to find a house.

Then I came to one place at the end of a row of dwellings less demolished than most of those that I had seen. It was the most difficult of all to enter because nettles and thistles had seeded themselves and grown up into a barrier which entirely filled the small, walled court at the side of the house. Nevertheless, that powerful instinct which tells travelers where they should or should not stay, instructed me that that was to be my house of all houses in Galilee! I therefore sought around for a long stick and with that I beat my way through the barricade of pricking weeds to the house door, which stood open. Beyond the court was only one room; it was partly roofless, and without a window, there being now a big breach where this had been dynamited out of the wall. That window looked once towards a view of absolute loveliness: the pointed heights of the hills of Syria, the River Jordan flowing below and away to the right again to that lake which God made for his delight – the Galilee.

I remember very well that as I looked down upon the lake through the broken wall of the house – my house – the lake, because of the heat mist floating over the water, was silvered and mauve-colored, so that it resembled a stretch of the autumn crocuses which clothe the foothills of Galilee at summer's ending.

Outside the window-place a eucalyptus tree shimmered and whispered in the way of that tree, which trembles with excitement even before the wind reaches its sensitive foliage.

The widening of the window site during the demolishing of the Arab houses had improved the room, bringing more light into the old place, and making it look less cave-like. The house was built of stone, pieces of crudely hewn rock cemented with mud. The earth floor was ankle-deep in crumbled plaster. Without further delay I went out to get a sweeping brush and pails of water. As I cleared away I found things left behind when the former occupants had fled across the Jordan into Syria. Several of my finds were touching. There was the child's riding-boot, almost doll-size, with a miniature, but sharp, spur attached; bunches of herbs, yet quite fragrant, one primitive earring of twisted wire hung with round blue beads against the evil eye. The earring I attached to Fuego's collar; he lost this protective charm some time later, and immediately met with a terrible accident. I found also many broken pots of attractive natural colors, many small primitive hand instruments for fieldwork, and also a great millstone. On the wall by the door was a rusted fodder rack, with dusty, dried maize leaves within.

I felt that I had come to what had once been a happy home, for the past owners had been fellow herbalists, and riders of horses, and had chosen to live alongside their horses inside their home, as do many Arab people, especially the Bedouins. The Bedouin women will even suckle at their own breasts the puppies of their favorite Saluki greyhounds to make their dogs more passionately attached to their households. The bunched herbs which I found amongst the rubble, judging from the scent of them when I rubbed them between my hands, were chamomile (*Matricaria chamomilla*) for the treatment of the ailments of babies, sage (*Salvia officinalis*) for wound cure, mallow (*Althaea officinalis*) for bruises, and the tassel part of maize (*Zea mays*) cobs [corn silk], found pressed into a big bunch, being a well-known Arabian remedy for kidney and bladder troubles.

Having swept up the rubble into two great mounds, I decided not to spade all of it up into buckets for removal, but to keep two small mounds at each end of the room where the floor was reached by window light, and there plant flower seeds. I usually have flower seeds with me as I travel: they make good presents. I had left with me, in my luggage, marigolds, sweet peas, and evening-scented stock.

As soon as the room looked in quite good order, I emptied the last of the numberless buckets which I had carried from the horse trough, my nearest water-supply, and planted my seeds. I was as dusty-looking as any miller, and painfully tired, for I had worked without rest, wanting to sleep in my Galilean house that same night of my finding it. Many times when depression at the enormity of my task had possessed me, I had only needed to go to the window place and look down upon the beauty which was mine whilst I lived there, to have my hands very willing again.

I made a table from the big millstone which I balanced between two rocks. As I moved one of the rocks into a more level position for better balancing of the millstone I discovered a nest of black scorpions! There they were, already formed in their peculiar yet attractive scorpion shape, with their young tails raised over their backs in stinging position at my disturbance of their dwelling-place, only they were at that time little larger in size than honey bees.

My first instinct was to pick up a stone and crush those dangerous creatures. I knew there were scorpions on the kibbutz lands; there had been much talk about them during our melon harvesting, how a sting from a yellow scorpion can kill a man speedily, so that the Arabs frequently cut off the limb immediately they have been bitten, cutting above the sting when possible, to prevent the dangerous poison from traveling to the heart. The sting of the black scorpion is not usually fatal but it "makes strong men cry," it is said, so that morphine must be given. However, I remembered the Talmud story of Rabbi Judah I, and the young weasels, and I decided to let the black scorpions live where I had found them. I felt that it was unlikely that they would sting me; they were yet young and I expected that I would have continued my travels elsewhere before they reached adulthood. Their parents were a different matter and I hoped that I would not meet them!

Finally I went outside my house, into a vermilion Galilean sunset, to gather herbs from the hills to bank in corners of my house and court, and make the place more pleasant. I cut also an amount of eucalyptus which was then in flower. This flower has a most pungent and attractive scent, and the swarming bees around eucalyptus trees drew my attention to this fragrance, as they have to many other tree blossoms. The Arabs now call the eucalyptus the "Jew's Tree" because the Jews have planted so many in Israel, one of its uses being that mosquitoes do not like its vicinity; it also gives excellent shade. I think that the rich-tasting and fragrant honey obtained in Israel, from the crowding blue-painted bee hives, is as much scented with the blossom of eucalyptus as it is with that of orange trees.

The doctor was brought to see my house, and it was approved, and I was promised a lamp and a bed; that was to be my furniture. I would be able to get several wooden boxes also! Only, when the two kibbutz members arrived

Summer in Galilee

with the promised things, they did not approve, and indeed were shocked at my choice of house. For they declared that the window gap directly faced the Syrian frontier and therefore, I could not possibly light a lamp at all within the dwelling, for it would show the hostile Arabs that that lonely outpost was now occupied. They said further, that the River Jordan, at that point beneath the house and for a distance along either side, was very shallow and could easily be waded by the Syrians. Finally it was believed that the Arabs from the village of which my chosen house was part, were in hiding in river caves in the near area, awaiting any opportunity to return.

I said that I would continue to live in the dwelling which I had chosen and cleaned with much hard work, and I would not burn a light. Stars are bright in Galilee in summertime, they had better take the lamp away so that I would not be tempted to use it.

Soon I became used to lying in my bed in the darkness with the stars to afford some dim lighting. I always slept out in the court, for although the house was as cool as any cave by day, it was oppressively hot by night when the stones, and even the earthen floor, threw back all the sun-heat which they had been absorbing from sunrise to sundown.

For my bed I was given only a thin hay mattress and one narrow sheet, as bed coverings were in short supply. I used new paper as an under-sheet, a towel where my face lay, and my dressing-gown to hold the top sheet in position. Often as I entered my bed at night, in its strange surroundings, I would say lines from the poem *The Wander-Light* by Henry Lawson (1867–1922), an Australian poet:

> For my beds were camp beds and tramp beds and damp beds,
> And my beds were dry beds on drought-stricken ground,
> Hard beds and soft beds and wide beds and narrow,
> For my beds were strange beds the wide world round.

The court of my house was small and square, with high walls. Only the walls were not high enough to prevent Fuego from going over them if he wished, for Afghan hounds are remarkable jumpers. This ancient breed from the mountains of Afghanistan possesses peculiar hind-quarters; the list of show points of this breed describes: "hind-quarters shaped like a gorilla." Thus the hound's tremendous spring. I did not want Fuego wandering alone in the surrounding hills by night, where he might be a victim of a jackal pack, or one of the huge serpents said to dwell there. He had run off once in to the wilderness of Galilee when he was young; a rattling can had frightened him, causing him to race away in panic. I had had to cut off the long silken hair which grows, mountain-goat-like, on the Afghan breed, using sheep shears in order to remove the tangled pieces of the barbed and thorny vegetation through which the dog had plunged in his sudden fear.

Now he was older and bold enough, and liked to chase the hares and wild turkeys to be found sometimes in the hills. He had not yet met with a snake; they had only been heard as they slid away, but he had been attacked by either eagles or giant buzzards in daytime when walking with me on the lonely and beautiful Emek hills some distance from Galilee, where Saul had consulted the Witch of Endor. Two enormous golden birds had swooped down out of the sky, despite their size unnoticed until their swoop. The hound, some distance ahead of me, had instinctively flattened himself upon the ground, keeping his head between his forepaws. The great birds had flown at his head, but missed their mark in the dog's sudden flattening of his body. Before they had mounted the sky again sufficiently high for their next plunging attack, I was at my dog's side. I frightened away the birds merely by pulling off and waving my bright red shirt at them. The birds hovered over my dog and me for a while, and then, as if in agreement, suddenly veered away at a great speed towards a distant ruin of a Crusader fort, which was probably their dwelling-place.

Therefore, from dusk until dawn, to prevent Fuego from leaving the court as I slept in the night, he was tethered to the foot of the iron bedstead. The doorway out from the court onto the hillside I kept barred with the use of a heavy wooden, iron-riveted door which I had taken from a neighboring ruin. There also was a large tunnel-like place to one side of the court, which led into and linked up with all the ruins behind. It was high enough for a man to come through. Over this place I made a barricade of wooden planks and boxes and many boughs of eucalyptus, the latter being renewed frequently as their leaves withered and fell. Anyone

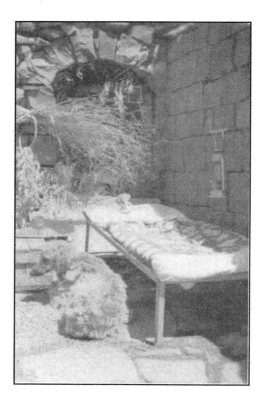

Court of my Arab house in Galilee

attempting to enter the court through that barricade would certainly be heard by both hound and me! And yet at night-time, when the stars were sometimes very dim because of the mists which rise from the near Huleh marshes, and there was no moon, it was that barricade which my eyes watched in apprehension.

I was pleased to have the company of the kibbutz horses and mules in their corral close by the back wall of my court. They were company in the night; I could hear the move-ments of them: shaking manes, pawing feet, snorting through the wide nostrils, indeed what the Gypsies properly call "horse music." Then, by day, I could enjoy their beauty.

In the corral was a striking Arabian mare of pure blood. She had been given in-foal to the kibbutz as a goodwill gift from their neighbor, the Bedouin Sheikh Abou Yussef. Her colt, now half a year old, was also in the corral; he was very wild. I was teaching him to drink water from a bucket. I called him in Arabic, *Howwah*, which means wind, because he snorted like a gale wind. Fuego was also friendly with the horses and mules, and sought their company. They would allow him into their corral and would not kick at him. In-deed, often in the daytime I would find him sleeping there, near the coolth of the water trough.

My friends in the kibbutz did not approve of my Arab house, and I was continually being warned of the dangers of such a place: of the scorpions which inhabit those old places, of the big snakes, and of the jackal packs which will attack if they find a lone person. Then, further, a trespassing Arab might pass by in the night and find me alone there! But my house possessed a fascination for me and I could not leave it. My flower seeds were growing fast on the rubble hillocks within the room. Seeds grow with such vigor in the dry heat of Galilee that one can almost watch them increase in front of one's eyes. The evening scented stock was in bud within a month, and the sweet peas were soon to bud. The marigolds made slowest progress, but they are flowers of the sun and there was over much shade for them within the house.

My court was a place for sun worship. No one could enter from outside without my agreement, and within the court I could bathe in the sun with a joy which was pagan. Sun is food for the human, rich liquid golden food which soaks into the flesh. The fears of the night melted away with the radiant sun of every morning, and the very first sights which held my eyes at every sunrise and filled me with contentment in my possession of my house in Galilee, were first: the Lake of Galilee as seen from my window, a golden harp then, always from the sunrise, not the Blue Harp which is one of the names by which it is known. And then: the sight of the kibbutz animals, the dark forms of the horses and mules in the corral, silhouetted against the shimmering primrose light of the growing sun, which would soon deepen the sky into the deep orange of marigolds. And always at that time the kibbutz sheep would pass by with Abel, their shepherd, coming up against the golden sky as they climbed the hill, the sheep the shape and gray-white color of a rain-cloud passing across the gold as they went to pastures distant from the kibbutz. The sheep were my reminder that it was time to leave my house and hurry to work in the melon fields.

The jackals of the area are so ferocious that at night lamps have to be hung around the fencing of the sheepfolds to protect the flock from jackal attacks; many a lamb had been carried off, and ewes and rams had had their throats torn out. I would be reminded of the safety of having a lamp in the night and my lack of one, when I heard the jackal packs howling in the dark, and that was very often. That jackals were near and numerous was evident from the melon fields. Jackals have a liking for ripe melons and they were very destructive to the crop, for they would go from melon to melon, merely taking out one mouthful from each, and they knew how to select with intelligence the best ones.

Bitten melons could not be used for fear of rabies infection. The marks of numerous jackal paws could be seen in the dust in the fields.

Then, one night, real reason for fear came to me in my Arab house. I was awakened nearly at dawn by the growling of Fuego. I turned to my dog and saw that he was watching the wooden door which barred outside entry into the court. Then I heard against that door the scratching sound of animal feet paws against wood. I left my bed and taking up one of the eucalyptus boughs, flung it against the door. The scratching was heard no more that night and Fuego settled into sleep. I felt sure that jackals had been out there. When it was light I searched around for paw prints, but could see nothing on the sun-baked and rocky ground.

Two nights followed without further trouble and meanwhile I rolled rocks against the door at dusk. Then came the climax! I was again awakened by Fuego in the night, but that time he was not growling but shrieking in a horrible blend of fear and rage, never heard from him before. Now my dog was facing towards the wall on the side directly opposite the head of my bed. There I saw a big dog-like form, as big as my own hound, far too large for a jackal, which is more the size of a fox. There were no dogs on the kibbutz lands other than my own, because they feared rabies from jackals. The animal on my wall was a grizzle color and its teeth were bared. The impression was confused in the night but I was made to cry out in real terror.

My cry sent the creature down from the wall and it ran off, for I heard the horses and mules stamping the ground of their corral in similar alarm soon after.

I now had to consider the distressing fact that neither my court nor the house was safe against the entry of the strange animal who had mounted on to the high wall and was therefore a climber. It seemed as if I would be compelled to leave my house. But I would have one more day and night there, for the following evening there was to be a kibbutz wedding and I would not return until nearly dawn, when there would be few hours left of danger.

I returned after midnight from the typical kibbutz wedding and it was full moonlight.

For the wedding the bride wore the white gown and veil which belonged to the kibbutz community and was altered there to fit each new bride. The groom and bride went straight from their work in the fields or workshops, after dressing, to be taken with their crowding friends in kibbutz wagons to the nearest synagogue. The only difference in the usual daily routine was that wine was served at table and a dance held through the night, with the noisy, stamping Israeli folk-dances predominating.

I had taken Fuego to safety with me, to the wedding dance, and on return to my Arab house, tethered him in the court while I brought water from the trough. Two of the kibbutz guards were on watch near the horse corral. I had warned them about the large animal. They told me that they had not seen or heard anything. Then, by the closed door of my house I saw a big dog. This, I thought, was Fuego. The only time that he was sure to play truant was at the time of the full moon. All Afghans are the same moon truants, as also are their closely related breed, the Arab Saluki. I moved forward then, very slowly, pretending not to see my dog, my gaze turned away, as I had learnt to do in catching wayward dogs and horses. The dog shape also began to move ahead, but slowly.

Only behold! that gait was not Fuego's! Fuego pranced; this animal ahead dragged its feet! It was the big, grimed intruder again!

On this occasion I was fully awake and I could see more clearly, it being full moon. The dog was of cattle-dog shape, more powerful than the greyhound build of Fuego. Its ears were cut off close to their base and the tail was cropped short.

I was moving forward faster than the dog, and when I was quite close to it, the dog unexpectedly stopped and turned to face me.

"Kelb! Kelb!" I called to the animal in Arabic. For it was surely an Arab dog [kelb] with its ears cropped so short. The Arabs often crop the ears off male puppies – to prevent later torn ears in fights when the dogs are older – and then feed the ears back to each puppy, the first meat on which the puppies are weaned. It is supposed to bestow the power of bravery on the dog to eat its own ears! Tails are cropped also.

"Kelb! Kelb!" I called again.

The dog came some steps towards me. It was certainly an ugly savage-looking creature, very well fed and powerful. Was it this creature which had been tearing out the throats of the kibbutz sheep?

The closeness of the dog caused me to feel interested, excited, and afraid, all at the same moment. Approaching noise of running feet was heard. It was the kibbutz guards who must have caught the sound of my calling voice.

The dog heard the men's coming. It lowered its eyes from gazing into mine. It had prominent, yellow ones. It turned then and began to move away again, not going in a fleeing panic; it merely trotted away. The guards asked me what I had seen and I told them about the dog. They said it must be followed and shot. I did not want the dog killed. I had called to the animal in friendship and it had delayed its going long enough, in answer to my voice, to endanger it. I told the guards that I did not know where the dog had gone. "It went into the night," was all that I could tell them.

They said that I had drunk too much wedding wine! Then, soon, we knew the direction of the dog. Up from the Jordan Valley there came a weird, heart-tearing, howling. Howling certainly, yet almost a love-call, then ending on a note of such extreme sadness it was like dying. There followed silence, until my own dog, startled at the sounds, started an answering barking. But no further sound came from the Arab dog.

Only by then I felt that I knew the history of that animal which had scratched at my Arab house door one night, and at a later night had clambered up on to my wall, frightening me. This was certainly the former cattle-dog of the Arab house in which I was living. It had probably been away from the home when its owners had fled, and had been unable to track them, as they had crossed water – the Jordan. Ever since, during two years, it had lived a wild, hunting life. It had certainly looked well fed. The outcast dog had sensed in some way that its former home was occupied, the home where it must have known happiness to have wanted to return. It had found there a stranger in possession and another dog in its place.

I felt convinced that that dog would never come home again. If it did I would try to retame it, and it could belong to a human as before.

The despair in the dog's howling troubled me. I thought about humans' stupid ways, how one race would hate another, often merely because their religion was different, or their marriage customs, or even eating habits. Innocent families were dispossessed and made homeless and the domestic animals suffered along with man.

The Arab dog was not seen again all the time that I was in the house, only something else came in the night – and it

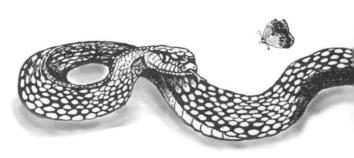

was a real danger this time – and fulfilled one more warning of kibbutz friends concerning the perils of living in such a place.

My dog awakened me again, this other night, with enraged barking, which was even more compelling than his warning when the Arab dog was on the wall. This time I was shocked to see a great snake coming towards my bed. I shall always remember the swishing sound of the creature as it came forward through the nettles and thistles from the part of the court which I had never cleared: it was like the quick scything of grass. Fuego was tethered as usual to one leg of the bed, to prevent him straying in the night, and he was leaping in rage at the oncoming serpent, which could well reach me from the head end without the dog being able to prevent this. And the snake's every intention seemed to be to attack me! This was extraordinary, for I had met with numerous snakes during my travels and all had fled as I approached.

This one in the Arab court challenged the baying, frantic dog, and moved closer towards the head end of my bed, its throat swollen with rage. I would not free my dog to have him killed very possibly, for the serpent was an enormous one: it stretched across the court. Its size, I think, accounted for its courage, although it is the small snakes (apart from the body-crushing pythons) which are said to be the most venomous; this one was no python.

I crawled quickly to the end of the bed where my dog was tethered so that we could then face the enemy together.

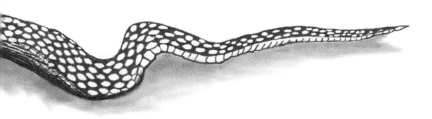

From there I flung at the snake the few things that I had around me, my sandals, some books, and finally my alarm clock. Only one sandal hit the creature. The glass of my clock shattered on the cobblestones.

How this would all have ended I cannot tell. I do not think that the snake would have approached the slashing jaws of my hound. The guards came then! They heard the commotion of my dog from quite far away. The snake fled, seemingly into the wall!

"What is it this time?" they asked. I told them about the snake and said that it was by the wall. At first they would not believe me, only they could hear from my voice that I was very frightened. I said that I dared not put my feet on the ground to cross to the barricaded door to open it, that I was too afraid. They said they would climb in through the window gap of the house. They came into my court with their guns pointed! I showed them the path that snake's body had made through the weeds in the court, and where it had entered the loose stones of the wall. Just then the snake put its head out from the wall. Quickly both guards fired at it. The dog had been barking throughout, although not so frantic now.

The shooting so near to him terrified him. I put my hand over his heart; it was beating like a wildly played drum.

The guards continued to shoot at the loose stones, but the snake could not be dislodged. Then it made its escape by the other side of the wall. I heard the animals in the corral stampede as they had done when the Arab dog had run past them, many nights since.

The guards reprimanded me and said that it was madness to sleep in such a forsaken place without a lamp. I told them that I had been forbidden one on first coming there, because of its nearness to the Syrian frontier. They said that I could burn a light in the court if I kept the house door shut. The high walls would hide any lamplight and with the door shut nothing could shine through the window facing towards Syria.

They brought me a lamp at once and I was never without it until I left the house. Only sometimes I forgot to fill it up with oil and it went out and the stars were dim, and I was in darkness again and awaiting the dangerous snake's return!

I had been told that one of the kibbutz bulls had been killed by a serpent and had its blood sucked. Also, soon after the snake's attempted attack upon me, from which my loyal dog had certainly saved me, the baker was attacked by a great snake on her way to the ovens. She had fled into the bakehouse with the serpent coming after her, "hissing like a steam-engine."

I always kept a stout wooden staff by my bed against the snake's return; my French friend Raoul had sharpened the end of it for me with his penknife, so that it was like a sword.

Raoul was a further reason why I delayed my departure from the Arab house. He appreciated the place as well as I did. He was not a member of the kibbutz, but was living there with a party of traveling workers who were building a vast silage tower. The building group was made up of workers from many lands in the typical Israeli way. Raoul was a French Jew, but of Algerian origin, his family being one of the silk-trading colony in Lyons. He had come to Israel four years ago and trained there as a builder. He spoke Arabic as well as French and Hebrew, and he was my first Arabic teacher in preparation for my planned visit to the Bedouin village of Toobah.

Raoul loved the Arab house; he delighted in the torn-out window view, and I have known him to stand there in silence for an hour. He liked the millstone table and appreciated the scent of the evening stock and sweet peas which had flowered exactly at the beginning of our friendship. He was the only person to whom I dared show my nest of black scorpions; they were quite big by then, but he agreed that they could not be killed. My dog Fuego had friendship for him, and would leap around the court in pleasure at his coming. I looked forward to my Arabic lessons when my work in the fields was over.

I had no covering for my floor of beaten earth within my house, and as I sat always on the floor, and my visitors did likewise, something was necessary. Therefore I used a large map of the world for a carpet. It was made of stout parchment and would not tear, and had traveled with me for years, but had not been used for floor cover before! This was folded up when not in use and spread on the ground only when required. Raoul and I, like two children, would sit on the countries of the world which we wanted most. All of Europe was his choice, from England to the far corners of Spain. I sat nearby on Turkey, with one hand over Mexico and the South Americas. I felt I could sit with surety on Turkey, for I was leaving for that country next, as soon as my work was ended in Israel.

The building of the silage tower seemed to be finished over-soon and Raoul went away. I was not so much in my Arab house after his departure. I lived mostly out in the court. Then the weather was cooling, as summer approached its always too-swift ending, and I wanted the sunlight more than ever. It was as if rat dwellers of the surrounding ruins knew that the Arab house was almost deserted again, for they came boldly one daytime and ate up all my flowers. Not a single flowering thing remained. The plants had been at the peak of their beauty then, and the scents of the evening stocks and the sweet peas had been a delight in the warm nights; even the marigolds had produced a few blossoms.

Like all the intruder animals which had come to my house in Galilee, the rats were very big ones. Soon after they had destroyed my plants, they appeared in impudent person one evening to knock over and drink a jar of milk which was my dog's chief food ration from the kibbutz. I saw a pair of rats run from the spilled milk as I entered my house;

they clambered easily up the rough stone wall, and balanced themselves on the few canes which were left of the former roofing. Those canes I vowed to cut down that very night.

The rats were abnormally big, the size of cats. They were ugly, with both long hair and an unpleasant smell. I would have left the Arab house forever the evening that I saw the rats, but it is said, and has often proved to be true, that troubles do not come singly, and that very week Fuego broke his leg. He had at that time lost the old Arab earring found on the floor of the house, with its blue beads of protection against the Evil Eye threaded on it; and the loss emphatically proved to be a bad omen.

My hound returned from his usual evening roaming over the near hillside, whining pitifully and dragging his right foreleg, which was so badly broken that little more than flesh held one broken part to the other. I sat on the ground and wept over my dog. I felt he could never survive his severe injury. I could not watch over him all the time. I would have to leave him for my work in the fields and to bring in our food; and in his lame state, serpent or rats would get Fuego. I remembered the paralyzed sheep which I had treated once on farms in the Pennine mountains of England; rats had eaten out their eyes in the night, so that I had insisted that if I was to continue to treat the sheep, lamps must be lit in the byres every night to keep away the rats. Most of the sheep had been cured with the help of herbs but many remained blind. Such doleful thoughts possessed me as I wept over Fuego, who himself had saved my life from the snake.

I had a friend Simon, of the kibbutz, who was a qualified veterinary surgeon, and I wanted his opinion as to whether the limb could be saved and his help in the setting of it if his opinion was favorable. For in my present demented state I was sure that I would set any limb crooked.

I tried to carry the injured hound up the hillside to the kibbutz, for it was already dusk, and I dreaded leaving him alone. He was far too heavy and the carrying pained his severed leg. Therefore I took him back to the Arab house, but left him outside there, within the corral of the horses, alongside the fencing. I felt that his friends the horses and mules would protect him for a while against the attack of jackals, rats, or anything else. Then I ran the whole way up the hillside, found Simon, and we ran the whole way down again, to the corral. Fuego was safe with the horses.

Simon looked at the terribly damaged leg and said that he thought it could be saved, as the dog was young and very strong. But I reminded Simon about the lack of good natural food for a dog in Israel, the impossibility of getting any raw meat, and how necessary good food was to make new bone. We decided to set the limb with cloth strips and wooden splints, no plaster being available. For my part, I do not like plaster; it prevents normal breathing of the pores, and is often harmful to the circulation, especially in a hot climate; therefore I did not regret its lack. Now I had to get Fuego away from the old house and court with all possible speed, as soon as his limb was set enough to enable him to be moved elsewhere. Simon had told me about a Turkish kibbutz on the frontier of Galilee, yet farther north, near to the River Dan. Simon knew also that I was in ill favor with the present kibbutz on account of my visits to the forbidden Bedouin village opposite, which had taken place at last. I went therefore to the Turks to ask if they had work for me, and told them of the handicap of my having a lame dog with me. They told me they were in need of a shepherd. As I had kept goats myself in England and had worked with sheep, and loved these animals, I accepted the work gladly. I was to spend there some of my happiest summer months in Galilee. I even discovered that I possessed a distant relative on my Turkish father's side in that kibbutz.

Therefore, one morning a week after my dog's accident, I was ready to leave my house. If it had not been for the rats

– which had become regular visitors to and fro along the roof cane edges, even after I had cut down all the remaining canes to thwart them – I would have regretted leaving the place very much. Since I had come to know the Bedouin Arabs, I had the added pleasure of their flute music on the hill across the valley opposite my house: and there is no sweeter, more compelling music played, no music more likely to make the listener want to follow after the player, than that of the piping of flutes; and the Toobah Beduoins were masters of such music.

Before I left I took a photograph of the court, with Fuego there, tethered to my bed, his cropped hair beginning to grow again (see page 150). At the head of the bed sat my talisman toy elephant. I lost the negative and retain only a small print to show how my court looked after I had cleared and cared for it through many months.

I was standing at the window gap, marveling at the always wonderful view along the Jordan Valley to the Lake of Galilee, and listening to the Bedouin flutes very loud and wild that morning of my departure, when one of the kibbutz mule-carts arrived helpfully to convey my lame dog up the hillside, and I went out through the court doorway for the last time, taking away with me memories which would remain always.

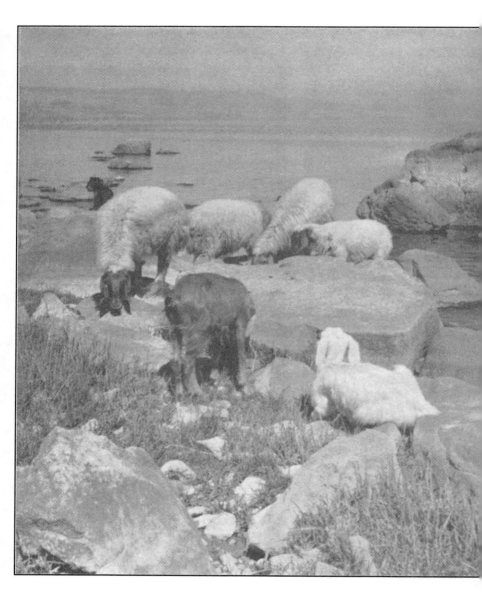

By the Lake of Galilee

Chapter Eight

A Bedouin Village

Travelers have said of Galilee that the farthest eastward shore of the lake is the end of the world that belongs to those-who-dwell-in-houses, and the beginning of that strange world of the black tents whose people spend their lives a-going to and fro over deserts. From the hills of Galilee right to the gates of Baghdad, they have possession.

Beit Sha'ar – house of hair – is a general name for the tents of black goat's hair of the desert dwellers; also, "the tents of Kedar" – the old Biblical name – is heard. One does not have to go that far beyond the Lake of Galilee to find the black tents. There is the big Bedouin village of Toobah in the hills above the lake, overlooking the Jordan Valley, and only a two hours' walk on foot from the old settlement of Rosh Pinah. There, in the hills of Galilee, live the Bedouin tribe of the powerful Sheikh Abou Yussef (see page 174), who has remained in possession of all his land despite the modern expulsion of most of the Arab families from the vicinity of the Lake of Galilee.

The village of Toobah remains strong in Galilee on account of the good services the Toobah Bedouins rendered to Israel in the Jewish War of Independence, when Toobah fought on the side of the Jews and proved to be skilled and brave fighters, and furthermore fed a large portion of the Israeli Army with the teeming cattle of Abou Yussef. I have met Israelis who fought in the war alongside the Toobah Bedouins who say they will always remember their valor. Sadly, it is said that now Sheikh Abou Yussef is a bitter, disillusioned man who feels that his people did not get either fair recompense for their services in the war or all that they had been promised.

All the time I was in the Rosh Pinah kibbutz near Toobah, the Bedouin village was forbidden territory to the kibbutz members because of ill feeling then prevailing between the kibbutz and Toobah on many counts, but especially because the Arab goat herds had eaten quantities of the young trees planted by the kibbutz. The village was further forbidden because it was under police investigation on account of alleged smuggling by the Toobah people of cattle into Israel from Syria and other Arab frontiers.

However, when I was in that kibbutz, it was unbearable for me to be living within sight of the interesting Toobah village which I longed to visit, and being prevented from doing so by "rules and regulations" which take over-much of the romance out of civilized life. As I was merely a temporary worker in the kibbutz, and not a proper member, I decided to defy the bans on my liberty to go where I wished – with the exception of the rule which banned being out alone in the countryside after nightfall. As for police regulations, I could pretend to be unaware of them.

Having decided to visit Toobah, my chief difficulties were that I spoke only the very little Arabic which I was learning especially for my visit, and that, being a woman, I had to have an escort, but none of the kibbutz members dared go with me. I could have asked my visiting worker friend in the kibbutz, Raoul, who spoke Arabic well, to take me to Toobah, but, as he was no mere visitor to Israel, he would certainly have been penalized if found there by the police, and I did not want that to happen. Therefore I waited my time.

One day, when I was working in the kibbutz fields below Toobah, harvesting garlic in place of the usual melons, a young man came from Toobah to buy garlic for the Sheikh's household. He wore ordinary European clothes, although jodhpurs in place of trousers, yet he attracted attention at once with the grace of his walk and his beautiful fine-featured face.

When leaving the field, the young Bedouin passed close by where I was working, and I got up from the ground where I was sorting out garlic, to tell him that I longed to visit Toobah. He looked pleased, his face smiling, and he put his hand on my soil-covered and garlic-smelling arm. "*B'vakashah*" ("With pleasure"), he said in courteous Hebrew, and told me further to be sure to visit his own family when I went to Toobah. "I am of the House of Abdullah," he said.

Soon after this visit, an English man visited the kibbutz. Marcus was only staying one weekend, but he promised to escort me to the Bedouin village. He spoke English and French, having lived for years in Paris. He was very elegant and I felt like a tramp at his side, with my sunburnt face and my frizzed and equally sunburnt hair.

I knew a woman in Rosh Pinah who told me once that Toobah women passed by her house daily on their way to and from a quarry where many of them worked. I, therefore, wrote a message in English to Abou Yussef, telling him that I was going to write a book about the Galilee and wanted to visit his village. One of his people from the House of Abdullah had said that I might do so, and I would like to visit Toobah on this coming Saturday morning. This message I left at the house of my Rosh Pinah friend, to give to one of the women of Toobah, for delivery to Abou Yussef. There was no post office delivery to Toobah.

Marcus and I set out for Toobah soon after sunrise, for we would be walking into the face of the sun most of the way, and we wanted to travel early before its full blaze. Also we were going the long way round, as we could not take the direct path up the hillside which faced the main buildings of the kibbutz since our visit was entirely forbidden.

Marcus again looked elegant in finely made French clothes and shoes of shining leather. I had taken trouble over my appearance and had hidden my weather-dried hair beneath my most brilliant scarf, which I had bought in Mexico. I also wore my best Turkish earrings, long ones of old ebony wood inlaid with gold. I was also wearing a properly ironed blouse and skirt instead of ones ironed only by the hot sun upon them after I washed them, which was my usual ironing method.

I know the fanciful thoughts that nomad men hold concerning women. Men who are a long time away from women, traveling in lonely places, from their very loneliness are creators of romantic ideas. I wanted to look at least a little like some of those ideas! I took my Afghan hound for the Bedouins to see. As they are lovers of fine dogs and horses, and the Afghan hound is closely related to the Arabian Saluki, I hoped they would like my dog. What was left of his cropped silken hair of a golden color had been brushed for an hour, and to my own appraising eyes the tall hound looked like an animal wearing a golden fleece.

Marcus and I hoped that the Sheikh had received my letter, for I had spoken with a German man and his wife who had been to Toobah once, and had gone there unannounced. They had met with closed tents; no one had spoken to them and they had been thankful to leave the place.

But I was already friendly with many of the children of Toobah whom I used to meet as they herded their goats by the old Arab cemetery, which I passed by frequently when I went to Rosh Pinah to buy white goat cheese for my dog –

there being no raw meat available for him in Israel. Those children at least would greet me.

When we had walked for nearly an hour away from the kibbutz, we at last came in sight of the first of a long stretching line of the black tents of the Bedouin. Ah! those tents of Kedar! The first that I had ever seen.

The big, black, hairy tents had woven awnings also of goat hair, of gray and black, and when we came upon them properly and saw how they crowded on the plateau on top of the hill in Galilee, they looked like a big company of cormorant birds sunning themselves, their wings outspread to dry after their water-diving, as I have often seen them do.

There were thronging children to be seen in and out of the tent doorways, lithe, brown-fleshed, with laughing faces, and gaudy clothes, and alluring as any mob of Gypsies! Big herds of goats skipped around, leaping from the gray rocks by which grew yellow-flowered thistles of sunflower form. I saw one family of goats which I considered to be the most magnificent that I have ever met, of pure type, black and tan, marked in the same peculiar way as the black and tan greyhounds of Afghanistan and Arabia. Hounds of both breeds I have bred and owned in England, from imported stock. There were fine horses also to be seen, tethered to posts by many of the tents. Wood fires glowed and smoke spiraled to the sky in tossing plumes of white and gray – to a sky which was already brassy with heat. But there was wind on that mountain plain where the black tents of Toobah crowded, the beloved *howwah* of the Bedouin Arabs, who themselves are often called "Children of the Wind."

One woman waved in friendliness to us from her tent door as we passed by. She was tall, aged, and had brilliantly hennaed hair, red almost as the fire embers, showing in curls pushing beneath her black headdress and falling on to her thin shoulders. Otherwise we continued our walk onwards without meeting with any person. Only the big Arab dogs, all of them mixed breeds, came leaping in fierceness at Fuego, whose own quick slashing jaws were well able to deal with his attackers; he was often too quick a fighter for my peace of mind. I thought frequently of the cold reception to visitors to Toobah about which the two Germans had told me.

We passed beyond the area of the tents, to where eucalyptus and pomegranate trees grew, and in their shade stood square houses of gray stone. Out from the first of those houses stepped a gray-bearded man, wearing typical Arab dress. He greeted Marcus and me, and told us that the Sheikh Abou Yussef was awaiting us in his house, and he would lead us there. I smiled happily at Marcus and we went onwards to the Sheikh's house, which looked much like the neighbor ones.

I had a present with me for Abou Yussef. It was an antique horse brass that I had found in an old saddlery shop in Yorkshire. It had the form of a camel within a crescent moon. I had bought it for my Afghan hound to wear, but it had proved too heavy for his young neck. He had been less than one year old when he came with me to Israel, to save me from the snake, and guard me valiantly all our time together.

I had been told by some people of the kibbutz who had seen Abou Yussef that he was a splendid-looking man, even now in his old age of possibly eighty years. His eldest son was also handsome, having been seen several times when dining in the kibbutz dining room on goodwill visits. It was also said about Abou Yussef that he was extremely proud and unfriendly, and would speak no word to his visitors, even when they came on special invitation. A Jewish general who now lives in retirement in a kibbutz by the Lake of Galilee, who had known Abou Yussef during the Jewish War of Independence, said of him that not only is he a philosopher, he commands also the power of being able to read the thoughts of all men accurately, merely by looking into their eyes. I was impatient for the immediate meeting with him.

The Sheikh's house seemed well built and cool. Outside the door was an assortment of footwear, from many tall and spurred riding-boots of typical Arab kind, with the pointed toe and wrought-iron heel, to sandals of mere canvas and leather thongs. I took off my sandals, which I saw that I had forgotten to polish! – this being out of keeping with the rest of my carefully prepared dressing for the visit, but more true to my usual appearance. Marcus put his fine, shining shoes next to my sandals. Fuego I tethered to the horse-post by the door.

Meanwhile, many Arab men had come to the doorway and were welcoming us. Within the house were gathered some twenty men. There were no women present. It would indeed have been an error of etiquette if I had gone to Toobah alone. I looked gratefully at Marcus, standing stiffly at my side.

Of all the men there, I knew instinctively who was Abou Yussef, apart from the fact that he was dressed differently from the others – he alone being dressed in black. He stood alone; king of them all! I felt that I was in the company of a remarkable presence. Abou Yussef wore a tight-fitting, long black tunic and a black over-cloak, all of a rich cloth. His hair, showing beneath his black, padded turban-form headdress was distinctly dyed black, though touched further with the red of henna, as also was his moustache and short beard. His eyes were outlined with kohl, dark eyes and fierce, and as they were directed into mine I felt that my soul was being searched! I could return the Sheikh's gaze fearlessly enough, for only admiration had brought me to his village, and the wish to write truthfully concerning what I saw there.

As I gazed back equally fiercely at the dark man, scowling in imitation of his expression, he put his hand across his mouth and laughed. With a wave of the same hand, he indicated to Marcus and me and the rest of the company, to be seated. Chairs had been brought for the visitors and Marcus sat on one. I sat on the floor where there were flat cushions spread, and the men smiled. I told them that I was as Arab and Bedouin as themselves in my ways, and conversation then began in a strange way, all of us seeking for words in Arabic, Hebrew, French and English. The Arabic words which I had carefully learnt from my friend Raoul in the kibbutz now proved to be of an Algerian dialect and were not easily understood. I decided that I would have to learn other Arabic if I were able to visit Toobah again. Some of the Arabs present were from, or had lived in, Damascus and Beirut, and knew a little French; others knew odd English words from their years in the Israeli Army. Therefore, altogether, until our departure, conversation never ceased.

Nor was Abou Yussef the silent, supercilious person described to me. He talked excitedly in Arabic and laughed like a boy. He spoke to Marcus and me through the other Arabs, and seemed especially pleased at my praise of his fine herds and horses. I told him of my admiration for his herd of black-and-tan goats that I had seen on my way to his house, and he agreed that they were some of his best. I said further that one day when traveling was over, and I had land of my own again in some country of hot sunlight, I would like to return to Toobah and purchase a pair of these goats. With typical oriental courtesy Abou Yussef said he would give them to me and I could choose a pair now if I wished. I thanked him but said that I found it difficult traveling with a large Afghan hound in modern transport, without taking a brace of goats around with me also! I would exchange a pair of young Afghan hounds when I returned for the goats.

The conversation then was of horses and dogs for most of an hour; Marcus's good French was a constant help. I told of my dog saving me from the snake; the Arabs said that they could be very dangerous. They asked me what I knew of the Arabian Saluki, and I informed them that they were being bred now from imported blood, in large numbers, in England and America, where they were highly prized, not only for their graceful beauty, but for their intelligent guarding of homes, and their gentle ways with children.

I asked, did they know of the verses written about the Saluki in *The Sacred Book of the East*, from the *Vendidad*, chapter 13. As they did not know them, and said they would like to hear, I recited in French, helped by Marcus, all that I could remember of the lines, though I was only able to quote fragments of the text, which I give here:

> He eats broken food like a priest; he is grateful . . . he wants only a small piece of bread . . . in these things he is like unto a priest.
>
> He marches in front like a warrior, he fights for the beneficent cow . . . he goes first out of the house . . . in these things he is like unto a warrior.
>
> He is watchful and sleeps lightly like a husbandman.
>
> He goes first out of the house . . . he returns last into the house . . . in these things he is like unto a husbandman.
>
> He sings like a strolling singer: he is intrusive, he is meagre, he is poor . . . in these things he is like unto a strolling singer.
>
> He likes darkness like a thief; he prowls about in darkness . . . he is a shameless eater . . . he is an unfaithful keeper . . . in these things he is like unto a wild beast.
>
> He sings like a courtesan; he is intrusive . . . he walks about the roads . . . in these things he is like unto a courtesan.
>
> He likes sleeping like a child: he is apt to run away . . . he is full of tongue . . . he goes on all fours . . . in these things he is like unto a child.
>
> If these two dogs of mine, the shepherd's dog and the house-dog pass by the house of my faithful people, let them never be kept away from it. For no house could subsist on the earth made by Ahara, but for these two dogs of mine, the shepherd's dog and the house dog.

Summer in Galilee

The Arab men and I – with Marcus close by on a chair – sat in a circle on cushions on the clean, tiled floor. In the center of the circle was the charcoal fire, possibly mixed with camel dung which gives a fierce heat when properly dried, for its crimson color opened out like a peony flower. Over it, coffee beans had already been roasted, and were being pounded with rhythmical music by one of the youngest of the men, using a pestle and mortar; it had made a background of sound like a distant drum to the Saluki lines.

The men were of all ages, several of them were fair-complexioned, with blue eyes. The most beautiful of them all had amber-colored eyes: pools of love in his exquisite

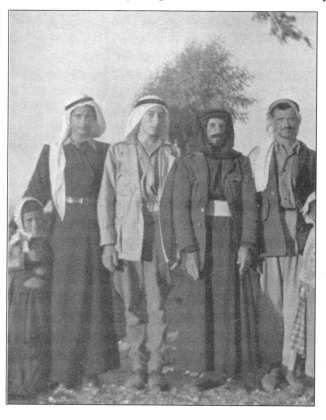

Sheikh Abou Yussef with Toobah Bedouins

face, I thought to myself. No man could ever have a more handsome face, and I expect he had already two or three Bedouin wives as beautiful as himself! He sat near to me and three places away from Abou Yussef. French-speaking, he had translated the Saluki poem into Arabic for Abou Yussef: his Arabic words had sounded like a lilting song compared to the shorter, slower ones of my spoken French.

Among the Bedouins of Toobah are families of black Arabs. They did not seem to marry with the lighter-complexioned Bedouins, for the many black children that I saw as we passed the tents, and also had noticed keeping the Toobah herds in the fields, were of a very distinctive type. Formerly I had met with several of the black Arabs when shopping in Rosh Pinah, and they had all been of massive build, a very different type from the slender graceful Bedouins. It is a fact that Bedouin Arabs have black slaves to serve them, but the Toobah Negroes must long have been made free men, for they and their children walked around with proud bearing. The black Arabs were now represented in the circle of men by two of their kind; one of them had wiry locks of gray hair showing beneath the white cloth of his *keffiyeh* headdress. They were interesting men. Not of African type, theirs were strange horse-like faces, with powerful and long noses, and long jaws, their eyes rolling and bloodshot like those of savage stallions. They spoke only Arabic. They sat close to the Sheikh and both seemed to be men of position, and proud of character.

The rich scent of the roasted coffee, now boiling, began to fill the room. The brass coffee-pot was put on the floor and more and more men came in to join the circle. Among them was one wearing dark glasses; he had been with the Israeli Army for a long time and could speak English better than the others could speak French. Now we had an efficient interpreter for all our languages, and Abou Yussef said he was very pleased to have him with us.

Coffee was passed to Marcus and me and the Sheikh, and then to the other men. Watchful, I saw that the black Arabs were served amongst the first, and I was pleased. We drank the coffee from fine porcelain cups of eggshell frailness, patterned all over with a veining of many colors, and gold, but without handles. Marcus said to me afterwards that he was tempted to hide his beautiful cup in his pocket handkerchief and carry it away with him! The coffee had the faint flavor and fragrance of coriander seed, which was delicious.

Conversation progressed better than ever over the coffee, with the fluent interpreter present. We spoke again about the Arab horse. The Arabs said sadly that motors and tractors would banish horses from the world; they cited modern Israel as an example, with its tractor-dominated farming. Marcus and I assured the Arabs that the death of the horse was yet far distant. Indeed there was a growing movement in many countries to bring back the horse and plow; farmers are insisting on cultivating their land by ancient natural methods. The tractor, with its heavy weight, presses the life and vitality from the topsoil of the earth, and necessitates the use of dangerous artificial chemicals which were like drugs instead of true foods for the soil. I would never allow a tractor on any land that I might own.

I said also, concerning the Arab people themselves, that come what may in the future, whatever senseless wars might be fought between others and themselves, I could never cease to admire them on account of what they had given to the world in their unexcelled horses and dogs, their delicate poetry, and immortal old palaces – and what would Spain be like without her Moorish palaces and flamenco singing and music! – and the ancient medicine of Avicenna which I, as a herbalist, closely studied and followed. The Arabs were pleased with such talk. But it was not flattery. I spoke with sincerity; I belonged in my heart to the same "backward" way of life as their own, and I wanted no change.

Sitting on the floor of the cool stone house in the company of Abou Yussef and his people and my sympathetic escort, I passed a morning to remember with pleasure and nostalgia always. When we had had three cups of coffee, Marcus and I discussed the matter of leaving. He had been as happy with the Arabs as I had been. For my part I would gladly have stayed at Toobah for the rest of my life! But we did not want to make the error of remaining over-long on a first visit. Marcus therefore told Abou Yussef that we must return to Rosh Pinah. Abou Yussef took our hands: "Come again to my house," he said. "Be sure to come again."

I thanked him in Arabic. That, at least, was something that I had learnt to say correctly. Laughing, he said farewell in Hebrew: "Shalom" (peace!).

I then gave to him the old horse brass, telling him that it was for a favorite horse to wear. His eyes softened with pleasure and he handed it round for the other men to see.

Before going out of the house I shook hands with each of the men, including the fierce-looking black Arabs, and the beautiful one of the amber eyes. "I'll never forget you," I said. I felt a deep sympathy for them all.

"Come again to Toobah," Abou Yussef repeated.

Marcus and I went out into the shimmering sunlight. I saw that my dog had been given a dish of water. The Arabs gathered around the Afghan hound, comparing his features with that of the Arabian Saluki. They asked me if I would unleash the hound so that they could see how he moved. I accordingly freed Fuego from the leash and he went racing out from the shade of the eucalyptus tree which sheltered the horse-post from the morning and early noon sunlight, and away over the plain with a pack of barking Arab dogs at his heels. But as he was the only one of the greyhound breed amongst them, he soon outpaced his pursuers, and making a wide circle, returned to my side. The Arabs shouted their dogs away and praised the swiftness of the Afghan hound.

Summer in Galilee

As Marcus and I passed by the tent of the henna-haired woman, who had waved to us previously, we saw her waiting outside her tent. She called to us, inviting us to enter her tent. We were pleased to enter there, and our hostess spread bright colored cushions on the floor for us to be seated. She insisted that Fuego be brought into her tent also, as the hound was panting from his running in the heat of the sun. Then she returned to her work at a hand-loom. I could see that the Bedouin woman was very old, her face patterned with the deep wrinkles of old age. Surely in her young womanhood she had been a beauty, with her glittering green eyes and her finely modeled face. Her face was tattooed with peculiar markings in indigo dye, general to most of the women of Toobah, and the same markings are seen also on the gravestones of the Arab cemetery at the foot of the hill on which stood Toobah. I was not sure what the marks represented. They looked to me like a V-shaped flight of birds or perhaps emblematic fir trees. In the case of our hostess, aged skin so distorted the tattoo marks that it was difficult to distinguish the pattern intended. Her hair was dyed so bright it was almost the color of a corn poppy, and was frizzed beneath her black headdress. This frizzed hair gave her almost an artificial look, quite like the figurehead of a ship.

I liked her instantly. She was the dramatic type of person that appeals to me. She sat on the ground by us and worked at the hand-loom on which she was making the coarse goat-hair fabric used for the outer awnings of the Bedouin tents. Her loom was simple, merely a square wooden frame fitted with taut strings. She thrust the coarse lengths through the strings, and then with a wooden peg-like instrument hammered the thread firmly down into the body of the material already woven. She swayed her tall, thin body to and fro in rhythmic motion as she worked.

The Bedouin made a good picture of primitive womankind at her loom. Her clothes were of the traditional Bedouin style: black, with touches of color, especially in the bright bands of material sewn one above the other at the hem-end of the ankle-length skirt and around the base of the wide sleeves. The *hatta* (headdress) was unlike the flowing muslin *keffiyeh* of the men, being of heavier cloth, and more padded, and of flat turban-shape, black with colored bands. She wore an ample supply of bracelets of silver and of colored glass, many finger rings, including several beautiful ones of wrought silver, big hoop earrings which tossed against the fuzz of flaming hair, and several necklaces. There were tassels of gold thread hanging from the broad sash belt of her gown. Her feet, of fine shape, were bare. With so much jewelry upon her person she made her own orchestra, sounding like jingle bells and cymbals; I feel sure she herself enjoyed the music of her person as she worked. She talked to us in high, shrill Arabic, comparing the good climate of Toobah on the hill plateau with that of the stifling heat of the land below.

"Here we have wind, wind," she exclaimed, speaking the Arabic word – *howwah* – with special love in her voice. "Come and live here," she told me. "You seem like one of us. Stay in my tent with me."

The skilled weaving of the woman and the primitive, yet artistic, cloth that she made were a joy to my eyes, as were also my present surroundings of the wide black tents with the sides flapping in the mountain breeze, the magnificent black-and-tan goats grazing around the tent door, and the view over the Jordan Valley to the Lake of Galilee, and all about us the strange music of the Bedouin camp; even the grunts of the many camels of the Bedouins could be heard.

We were not long alone in the weaver's tent; young girls and children began to enter within, or gather in the doorway. They were not dressed in black like the weaver, but were as gaudy as the king birds of Galilee which eat bees, and they jingled like Gypsy girls, wearing as much jewelry as the weaver, and even more than her, for many of the girls had further ornaments bound into the ends of their long black hair, which they wore either free flowing or plaited.

Some of the older girls came close to me and touched my face with their hands, and commented that my skin was as brown as their own. They stepped lightly across to Marcus also and touched his college tie, wondering at it, for it seemed that they had never before seen a man wearing a tie! Each time that he moved they fled away like butterflies, only like butterflies to settle close by again!

Marcus began to distribute coins. That gave so much pleasure that I am sure he entirely emptied his pockets and deprived himself.

One of the girls was of especial beauty and other eyes seemingly had appraised her, for alone of her companions she wore costly earrings and a silver stud in her nose, pressed through the right nostril. She was very straight and tall, and dressed in a long close-fitting dress of a rich orange-red material, so that her small pointed breasts looked like the buds of pomegranate blossom when ready to open into flower. Her skin was not as dusky as the others, but was the color of old ivory with its shading of cream and brown, and the delicate carving of her face and arched neck was again like finished ivory. I felt sure that she had been chosen already in her childhood as a bride for one of the Sheikh's sons.

I told her how beautiful I found her and she laughed in pleasure, hiding her face in her hands in a Gypsy-like gesture, with her dark and brilliant eyes smiling at me through the ivory window bars of her fingers, the tips of which were each touched with the red dye of henna.

Finally we had a visit from apparently one of the great ladies of Toobah, for all the children and maidens either bowed or kissed her hand as she entered the tents and those around Marcus fled from him. She was past middle age, of big stature, and her body was heavy with pregnancy. Her clothes were similar to those of the weaver, but of richer stuff. She had silver and gold threads shining in the cloth of her black headdress, and on the back fall of this were rows of small golden tassels. Big gold ornaments rested on her heavy breasts, and round the lower part of her body was wrapped a finely embroidered shawl, having a design of palm leaves, the shawl so wrapped as if to support the embryo child that the woman held within her. Her face was heavily tattooed in indigo dye and her eyes darkened with kohl. Her face was pallid and fat, but her eyes flashed in beauty of that amber color which I so much admired earlier that morning, and her bearing was high caste. The weaver treated her with the same deference as shown by the girls and children.

The great Lady of Toobah stayed with us for some ten minutes. She mostly stood staring and smiling, for conversation with her was more difficult than it had been with the weaver, with whom we had spoken much through laughter-provoking signs and gestures. Finally she said farewell, and that she was on her way to the Sheikh's house. Marcus and I then also told the weaver that we must leave her and she asked us to stay longer and share her meal, which she would soon be cooking. But we were firm that we must go. At her tent door she hugged me to her, stroking my face and saying that she would remember me as tenderly as any daughter. I replied that I would remember her as a mother. And surely she would have been a good mother for anyone to have, with her warm-hearted manner and her sense of humor.

Most of the young people also touched my face and Marcus's hands as we passed out of the tent into the noonday sun. Then a group of small boys, including several of ebony skin, accompanied us down the road. I gave one of the boys my dog's leash to hold and he was joyful. That was a sight to see, the little dark child in a striped shirt of yellow and red, with baggy trousers of sun-faded green, leading the prancing, shaggy, golden dog over the hill ridge.

Summer in Galilee

At the foot of the hill, where the Toobah road joined the main one to the kibbutz and Rosh Pinah, we met a large herd of goats and fat-tailed sheep coming towards us with bells ringing, and there was also the sound of shepherd flutes. The sun burnished their healthy bodies, and I watched their advance with admiration, even though they did cover me with dust.

With the herd came a group of young Arabs who greeted the children with us, and then I saw at the rear of them all, the son of the House of Abdullah. I had looked for him amongst the people of Toobah but had not seen him. We talked with him for a while in our limited Hebrew and I told him a little of my impressions of Toobah, and my admiration for Abou Yussef. He then repeated his earlier invitation which had certainly helped me to get to Toobah. He said: "When you return to Toobah, be sure to visit the House of Abdullah. My family were expecting you this day."

I promised that I would do so and thanked him again. I did not know then in what difficult circumstances I was to fulfill that invitation.

The Arab boy politely gave me the leash of my Afghan hound, and then the children who had come with us joined the group with the flocks. The flutes were played again and the whole party moved away up the hill to Toobah. I wished that I was going back to Toobah with them that very hour.

Soon after my return from Toobah, I came to know an Arabic-speaking Jewish worker from Iraq who had come to the kibbutz as the chief of a team of workers employed to clear more of the kibbutz fields of stones in order to make tractor cultivation possible. He stopped me to admire my Afghan hound and spoke to my dog in what seemed to be excellent Arabic. I told him that I greatly wished to learn to speak good Arabic; it had been my mother's first language as she was Egyptian-born, from Alexandria, and spoke Arabic more easily than European languages, which she also knew. He said that he would give me Arabic lessons in exchange for English lessons from myself. I agreed readily.

Like many people from Iraq he spoke fairly good English already, also Hebrew. His name was Leo. He looked more like a small hairy monkey than a lion! He knew about my visit to Toobah; many people in the kibbutz had come to know, though as yet I had not been officially reprimanded. Leo told me that he was planning a visit to Toobah himself, as he spoke the same type of Arabic spoken there, and that he would take me with him when he went. I felt that he would be a most helpful interpreter if he could speak the Bedouin Arabic, and also English. I told Leo to advise me several days before his planned visit to Toobah, as I wanted to send a courtesy letter previous to the visit, especially as I wanted to have photographs of Abou Yussef and his village, and would not like to take my camera there without having notified the Sheikh. I remembered the careful etiquette experienced on my first meeting.

Leo proved a difficult teacher of Arabic as he wanted to marry his pupil! That was no great compliment to me; there were so few women in Israel at that time, compared with the numbers of men flocking into the new state, that marriage proposals were easily come by. I avoided that one by stating firmly that I already had a fiance, that I was leaving Israel for Turkey very soon, and had no intention of marrying anyone at present. Leo's reply was that he intended to marry me within one month, that his age was approaching forty, and his family had long been telling him that he must marry. He had already written his family that he had chosen a wife who looked and lived like a Bedouin Arab!

Although I was reluctant to do so, I decided to end the Arabic lessons, being by then able to speak some elementary Arabic quite easily. I still wanted to go to Toobah with the Iraqi Leo as interpreter, but a month went past and no visit was arranged. Then, I met in Rosh Pinah one of the

French-speaking Arabs who had been present in Abou Yussef's house when I had visited. He asked me when I was going to return to Toobah, as many of the Bedouins there were looking forward to seeing me there again. I replied impulsively that I would go to Toobah that coming Saturday morning, that I would confirm this by formal letter, and meanwhile would he give my regards to Abou Yussef and all whom I had met at Toobah who had made my visit such a happy and interesting one.

On my return to the kibbutz I went at once to the place where Leo's tractor team was working, and told him of my meeting with the Bedouin, and that I was going to Toobah that coming Saturday. Would he escort me there as promised? And write me the formal visiting letter in Arabic as he had also promised? He had told me that before coming to Israel he had been a visiting teacher in Arab village schools around Baghdad. Despite his rejected marriage proposal and the ending of the Arabic-English lessons, I had remained on friendly terms with him and often brought him bruised, rejected melons from the melon harvesting where I was still working. They were good eating if consumed at once, and being from Iraq he had a great liking for melons.

He promised to take me to Toobah on Saturday, and came to my house that day to write the required letter in Arabic. I told Leo to write that I wished to make a farewell return to Abou Yussef and Toobah on Saturday morning, that I would like to take photographs for my book whilst at Toobah and would bring my camera, and that I remembered my previous visit with gratefulness and pleasure. The letter written, I signed my name. It was a joy to see the picturesque Arabic writing, and I felt that it was a compliment to Abou Yussef to be sending him a letter in his own Arabic without necessitating translation from my English as before. I sent the letter the same way as my first one, by the quarry workers from Toobah, who passed through Rosh Pinah. Leo promised to be ready to leave with me soon after sunrise, as Marcus and I had done previously. Marcus had returned to England a few days after our happy visit to Toobah.

In readiness I purchased a large supply of sugar sticks of all colors and fancy wafer biscuits for the Bedouin children who had been such delightful company, and I made my camera ready.

On Friday evening Leo came to tell me that he had to go to Haifa for the night and therefore would be unable to take me to Toobah until Saturday afternoon, when he would certainly return. I was angry with him, telling him that I never failed to keep my promise to anyone, and it was too late to notify Toobah in time for the Saturday morning. They would be expecting me and I would not arrive. It was tragic!

Leo replied that the change of plans was unimportant, that he knew the Arab people far better than I did, and that time meant nothing to the Arabs. I was not so sure; I remembered the careful courtesy and formal etiquette shown by the Toobah Arabs on my previous visit. Saturday afternoon came and went without the return of my escort. I was overcome with shame on account of my rudeness shown to Toobah, although the fault was not mine.

I went to the tents where the tractor team lived and asked for news of their chief. I was informed that Leo had gone to Haifa for the whole weekend!

Sunday morning came, and went also, without the return of my escort, and I promised myself that without question I would go to Toobah by myself if the Iraqi man had not arrived by the mid-afternoon.

Meanwhile I went to see a good Greek-Jewish friend of mine who was staying temporarily at the kibbutz. She was not Arabic-speaking but had traveled much in the Middle East with her husband, a pearl merchant, and she knew the Arabs quite well. I told her how desperate I felt. She told me not to worry, that I had said that the Toobah Sheikh was a shrewd philosopher and able to read men's minds; therefore he would know that something had kept me away from Toobah and that I would be sending him an explanation.

"You cannot go there by yourself," she warned — herself reading my thoughts. "That is impossible."

Only I was not so sure that all was as well as my Greek friend assured me. There were those flutes of Toobah; they sounded angry! I was used to the Toobah flutes in the hills piping their herds to and from the village, or piping merely for the love of music. Since my visit they had seemed to pipe more often from the hillside across the Jordan Valley facing my Arab house — only it was possible to have imagined that increased piping. But the flute music all the Saturday afternoon and the following Sunday morning, when I should have been visiting Toobah, was loud and incessant, and angry — almost martial — and that was not my imagination!

I made myself ready to go to Toobah alone that Sunday afternoon, filled my old rucksack with the sweets and biscuits that I had bought for the Arab children, put in my camera also, and some Gypsy photographs of my taking which I wanted the Bedouins to see — but then stood in my doorway listening to the flutes and further delaying my going.

At that hour Leo came hastening down the rock path to my house. I was ready to condemn him in absolute anger for his churlishness, but he put in his words first. Without even having greeted me he shouted out:

"We can't go to Toobah now!"

"What do you mean?" I demanded.

"Three men have just been over from Toobah. They are very angry. The whole village is angry!"

"I should think so," I said, still hearing the martial flutes, although they were no longer playing since the past few minutes, and I did not hear them again whilst Leo was with me. I added: "I've never yet in my life asked for a meeting with someone and failed to arrive."

"But it's far worse than that," Leo continued. "Those idiots at Toobah can't read Arabic properly! They misread the letter that I wrote for you, and imagined that everyone from the whole kibbutz was visiting Toobah with you – a sort of goodwill visit to the end of hostility between them and Toobah! Therefore, Abou Yussef killed and cooked many sheep and bought large quantities of wine and fruits in the markets. They are very angry now, those at Toobah!"

Despite the hot sunlight upon me in the late summer noon, I felt my flesh chilling. Remembering the charm and delightful company of the Bedouins on my first encounter, and in contrast this insult inflicted upon them by me – the feast prepared and no guests arriving to take part in it! Certainly everyone in Toobah would be very angry!

"How terrible!" I exclaimed. "How really terrible. The only thing left for us to do to lessen this insult is to go at once to Toobah and apologize, and explain to them. Of course! Of course! Come on now. No more delay. Perhaps we can overtake those three men and return to Toobah with them. Let us run!" I continued: "Can you run? I can run very fast." Emotion was making me speak like a child.

"The men left for Toobah a while ago," Leo replied. "And we can't possibly go at all. They will kill us at Toobah."

"Not go!" I shouted. "Leave them there with their un-eaten feast and no explanation! The flies gathering on their goodwill feast!" I was trying to stir Leo's feelings.

"Come on," I cried, moving then along the path and calling to my dog, to put him on the leash.

"Come back!" Leo bade me. "I said already we can't go! You don't know Arabs. I know them. They'll kill us. And what's more they know that they can do that and go unpunished, for any court would agree that they'd the right to do so because they've been insulted. They'll not kill us on their village land, but as we leave it; that's the Bedouin way."

"The Arabs of Toobah are my friends," I said. "No man kills his friends, whether Arab or Jew."

"We can't go," he shouted. "Why, it's almost evening already. To be there after dark at any time would be crazy, but after what's happened now, it would be the end of both of us."

"All right," I said. "I'll go by myself. I'm going this very moment. Only I warn you, don't set foot near my court or house again, or it's not the Arabs who'll be killing you!" My voice raged. Then I began to run along the hill path.

I really expected that the Iraqi man would follow me. He was supposed to love me, judging from his repeated proposals of marriage! But looking back I saw him lolling against the wall of my court. Well, he would never loll there again as long as I occupied that place, I told myself, as I hurried onwards, my hound prancing at my side.

I had to go the long way round, along the same winding road that I had taken with Marcus. After what had happened I dared not go the direct way up the hillside facing the kibbutz. I feared that the kibbutz chiefs might stop me and turn me back. It was still forbidden to go there at all. Even if I ran they could easily overtake me on their mules.

It was a cold and lonely road, and I moved along it in misery. The evening breeze arose, blowing quite cold, for summer was ending. I shall remember the snake that I saw by the roadside resting on a rock near to where the other road commenced upwards to Toobah. It was the finest-looking snake of all that I had seen, in Israel or elsewhere. It was sunning itself in the last rays of the setting sun, absorbing into its body also the heat given out by the rock as it cooled in the evening air, a short thick snake, the lower half of its body coiled, the other part held upright with the sun touching its flat, triangular head. It was a distinctive silver color, with peculiar loose scales all over its skin, looking like the chain armor of medieval knights; there was a salmon-color shading on the silver, which was not of the setting sun. The snake must have heard the approach of my dog and me, some time before it left the rock, for we were running noisily. But it let us approach quite near before it slithered slowly down from the rock and disappeared within a thicket of thistles.

I turned up the path to Toobah then. The breeze blew chill around me and my hound, and the road was lonely and thronged with evening shadows. The armor-like scales of the snake had put me in mind of words of the Crusaders as written in Joinville's *Chronicles of the Crusades* – suitable words for the present journey to Toobah:

> He is ill-advised who, through fear of death,
> does what will be a reproach to him for ever.

We ran onwards.

I reached Toobah at twilight. The star Venus was early in the sky. I had passed uneventfully up the Toobah road and by the main body of the Bedouin tents on the plateau. No person had come forward to me; even the children seemed to be keeping within the tents. I had hoped that the weaver woman might be at her door and wave to me as before, but her tent remained as silent as the others. Only the angry barking dogs came out to my dog and me.

I found my way to Abou Yussef's house and tethered Fuego to the horse-post; then, having taken off my sandals, I went within, uninvited.

This time the Sheikh's house was filled with women and children. There was not a man present, but I saw the Great Lady of Toobah there, and she got up from a low seat of piled cushions and came to me, taking my arm in a friendly gesture. I shall always remember that my face was wet with sweat at the run up the hillside. There had been no heat left in the sun at the time of my leaving for Toobah, but my head-scarf and my hair pressing out beneath clung to my skin across my forehead. Perhaps the horror of the closed tents had increased the sweating; tents were habitually closed when the cool of the evening came at summer's ending. I shall always remember the Great Lady of Toobah, with the wide sleeve of her black Bedouin gown, wiping the sweat from my face.

They brought me water and small cakes, but I had no appetite for either and shook my head, thanking them. Then, using the little Arabic which I had learnt, first from my friend Raoul with pleasure, and then from the Iraqi man with great difficulty, I managed to make the Toobah women understand how ashamed and sorry I was concerning Abou Yussef's feast, and I wanted to find the Sheikh quickly and tell him this.

When the women saw that I was too restless to stay with them, the Great Lady said she would take me to Abou Yussef herself. I shook hands with all the women, nearly twenty of them. Then, by the doorway, I remembered the sweets I had in my rucksack for the children. I took out the many bags and opened the tops so that the children could see the bright colors of the sugar and biscuits, then I piled all upon one of the cushions and called to the children: "Come! Come!"

They came to the sweet things as quickly and noisily as bees winging to spilled honey. I heard the Bedouins laughing at the excitement of their children.

At the door, a young woman stopped me and said she would put kohl around my eyes to please Abou Yussef when I met him. She brought out from an embroidered bag a small circular silver box studded with bright beads, and also took out a flat piece of shiny black wood. I agreed to have my eyes painted with kohl, and she then dipped the stick into the black contents of the box and applied this around my eyes. The other women gathered around, laughing and exclaiming. No person in the Sheikh's house showed any anger towards me, only kindness and affection. I supposed the anger belonged to the men and would come later.

The Great Lady beckoned me to follow her. I took my dog's lead. She insisted on carrying my rucksack. I apologized that it was heavy, and showed her my camera within.

She told me that Abou Yussef was visiting at the House of Abdullah, and it was to there that she was taking me. The House of Abdullah! How strange. I was to go there after all.

That house closely resembled the Sheikh's: square and large and cool. Through the open door came men's voices. I left Fuego by the entrance. I had to tether him to a young eucalyptus tree, for the horse-posts were occupied by a trio of Arab horses. When I had reached the door I remembered that I still had kohl round my eyes. I showed this to my companion and she laughed very much and pushed me into the room. At the same time she indicated that she would be awaiting me at the door, and seated herself on the doorstep, her heavy body filling the entire entrance. From there she smiled at me warmly, as if to say that she stayed there for my protection and would not be leaving without me.

Abou Yussef was sitting on cushions on the floor in the company of four young men. The son of the House of Abdullah, known to me, was not there. But two of the young men resembled him and were surely his brothers.

I did not frighten myself by thinking of the anger that Abou Yussef must feel towards me. Taking off my sandals, I quickly crossed the room to him and took his hand. He asked after my companion, and I said I was alone with one dog.

He studied my face for some minutes, and I told myself in thankfulness that I really had done nothing wrong; the trouble had not been of my making. The burning, searching eyes would have terrified me otherwise. I then told myself that I had come all that way to apologize and had not yet done so. Therefore, I said, in Arabic, with great feeling:

"I am very sorry."

I could say no more. But he would know what I meant. Minutes of silence followed. The young men said nothing. One was pounding coffee. The scent of the freshly roasted beans was pungent in the room, bringing memories of my first happy visit to Toobah. All the time, Abou Yussef's powerful eyes searched my face. Then, abruptly, his eyes softened and, raising his right hand, he made a gesture of forgiveness, a quick wave from side to side of the slim dark hand.

"Forget," he said. And: "Think no more of this."

That way I was forgiven. My own eyes softened in admiration at the fineness of this man. He took my hand, gesturing to me to be seated on the cushion next to him. So now I was given a place of honor at his left side.

Still I wanted to explain further to Abou Yussef as to what had delayed me, and as to my letter having either been misread by the Toobah Arabs, or miswritten by the Iraqi man — perhaps deliberately as a stupid joke. I would never know. None of the men present could speak other than Arabic and a little Hebrew. Abou Yussef spoke only Arabic, and he was firm that no further word should be said concerning the mistaken feast.

Abou Yussef was still wearing festive dress and was even more striking than I remembered him on my first visit. How black his side pieces of hair and his moustache and beard had been dyed! His eyes were outlined darkly with kohl as before. Around his waist was a broad sash of crimson tussore silk. How fine he looked! And how much I loved him!

Seeing the kohl around his eyes I remembered again that mine were painted, and I pointed to my eyes and Abou Yussef laughed and called out to the Great Lady on the doorstep. She replied back to him, laughing loudly again, and we all laughed.

Meanwhile, outside the door of the House of Abdullah had gathered a great company of Arabs unlike anything that I had seen at the time of the visit to Abou Yussef's house. The sound of the people came into the room like a storm blowing outside. And that made me look towards the door, and I saw how the sun had set, and realized in sadness that it was too late to take photographs of Abou Yussef. I reached for my rucksack and took out my camera. Within its wide leather holder I had some of my best Gypsy photographs, hoping they would encourage Abou Yussef to let me photograph him, for I felt that the Gypsies were not far distant from the Bedouins, and that the Sheikh would like those photographs of the handsome people with their dogs and horses, tents and wagons (see page 196). Also, several of those pictures showed my own dogs, Arab Salukis and Afghan hounds, taken in company with Gypsies of many lands.

I was collecting my Gypsy photographs to illustrate a my lengthy book concerning life with the Gypsies, which book was to carry some lines of the poet Rimbaud:

> . . . walking slow
> Through Nature, I shall rove with Love my Guide,
> As Gypsies wander, where they do not know.

I had big enlargements of my photographs which showed well the beauty of the Gypsies and that look of untamed wild which is theirs. Abou Yussef was delighted and praised all and passed them to the young men, and finally they went to the Great Lady.

The young men questioned me concerning the Gypsies. "Bedouwi! Bedouwi!" they kept exclaiming. I replied to them as well as I could manage. They were charming, with laughing eyes and of type as finely made as their beautiful horses waiting by the door.

"Come," Abou Yussef then said, and pointed to my camera. I tried to explain that the photos would be poor ones in such a faint light, as it was then evening and Venus had been long in the sky above the eucalyptus trees and pomegranate bushes. More time was then lost whilst the Arabs were deciding who would be photographed. I suggested to Abou Yussef that he have the fine Arab horses as a background, but he disdained this proudly, as they were not his own.

I took only three photographs before the light went entirely. For two of these, Abou Yussef called to a stranger with a moustache to be photographed at his side, and to bring a child with him. I wondered if they could be a son and grand-son. As I took the photographs, I observed my hound in the background. Fuego looked entirely happy, sitting on his haunches, surrounded by an admiring crowd; again a deep dish of water was placed close by him.

I saw that it was now night. Darkness falls swiftly over Galilee, and while I still lived on the kibbutz lands I had a promise to keep: that I would not be out alone, beyond calling distance, after dark. The promise had been made to the kibbutz during my first week there, when one moonlit night, hearing the jackals howling for the first time, I had gone out searching for them. The guards had seen me far from the kibbutz buildings and had been angry with me, telling me that I was endangering them and others, not only myself.

After the few photographs had been taken, we returned to the house, where coffee was ready; it was served in fine porcelain cups the color of amber, and lightweight as amber. I pointed to the sky and told Abou Yussef that I could not stay longer. But he insisted that I drink one cup of coffee.

I then got to my feet and he, too, stood up, as did the young men. Abou Yussef told me that one of the young men of Abdullah would accompany me to the kibbutz lands. He suggested that I go back the quick way, straight down the hillside. I agreed to this. The kibbutz authorities would be angry with me already for my previous visit to Toobah, and then today's big trouble over the feast; a little more anger would make no difference.

Therefore, it was farewell. I would not be back for many years. I said goodbye, touching hands all round. I would have liked to kiss Abou Yussef's hand for all his gracious-ness to me. Only, lacking the courage, I shook hands, and embraced instead the Great Lady, still seated on the door-step. She kissed me warmly.

Many persons came forward from the doorway to shake hands. I finally gave Abou Yussef my Gypsy photographs, with which he seemed pleased. I also promised that I would send him copies of the photographs taken that evening if they came out at all.

I took my dog's leash, waved to all again and began the steep descent down the rocky hill path, accompanied by the young man.

Many people of Toobah gathered on the hill ridge and waved after us. I wished those of the kibbutz could have seen that sincere goodwill. How much better if there had been friendship with their Bedouin neighbors. I was aware that the Bedouin Sheikh had said to the kibbutz chiefs that his people, being Bedouins, were natural foragers, and might take away the kibbutz tools if they were left out in the fields. But Abou Yussef said also that, in time, they would become more disciplined. Meanwhile he would replace anything that they took.

The path to the kibbutz below had fallen into disuse. Dislodged hillside rocks made many blockages which forced us into the scrub of scratching thorns and thistles in order to traverse them. The young Arab lifted me over the worst places, and then went back and lifted my big hound to safety also.

The lights of the kibbutz below soon were quite close; the ground ahead became less wild and then we were across the frontier dividing Arab land from Israeli land and in one of the kibbutz maize fields. ("They'll not kill us on their land, but as we leave it," the Iraqi man had said.) The maize cobs were ripe and the leafage rustled pleasantly in the night breeze.

I gave the Arab my hand in thanks, and he, without any explanation, or asking word of permission, took me in his arms and kissed me. Then he went back to Toobah, and I went onwards to the kibbutz, unpunished by the Bedouins, and my affection for them so sincere that it would be a pleasure to write my memories of them and Toobah when the time came.

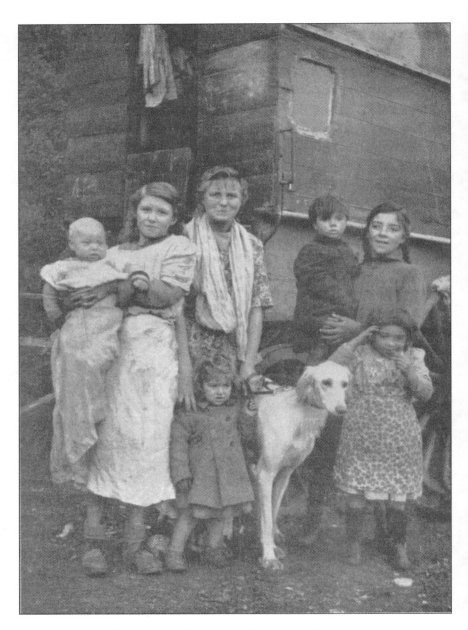

Gypsy wanderers on Banstead Downs

Chapter Nine

Shepherd in Galilee

Traveling with my lame hound from the Rosh Pinah kibbutz to the lands of the Turkish kibbutz of Hagoshrim took me to the far north of Galilee. The Hagoshrim lands are close to three frontiers, Lebanon, Syria and Transjordan. That part of Galilee was, for me, a new and an enchanted land, with its numerous coursing torrents – arising from mountain springs – watering fertile plains, and everywhere old Arab fruit gardens.

Some of the gardens had grown up into dense groves of fruiting things mingling with the wild oleanders, hawthorns, and water-canes; there the old vines, also turned wild, covered everything with their emerald braids and even mounted up into the highest boughs of the fig, peach, and walnut trees. Most of those fair gardens were deserted now, following the partitioning of Palestine, with their former owners away over the frontiers, and now landless refugees.

As a shepherd I had entry into the fruit groves, for there by the streams were to be found lush grazing for the flock of over two hundred sheep which I shepherded for the Turkish kibbutz.

One landmark of that area which is especially memorable was made by the Moslem Turks during their quite recent occupation of Palestine preceding the British Mandate. Where the mountain foothills formed an immense crescent moon, within the inner curve of that crescent, the Turks planted young oak trees in the form of a star. The oaks, being well planted – near to a perpetual torrent and pool of spring-fed water – achieved great girth and height. From an aircraft or a mountain-top, the star and crescent, emblem of Islam, can be seen plainly. It is appropriate that the first group of Turkish-speaking Jews, mostly from Istanbul and Smyrna, should have their kibbutz in that part of Israel. They called their kibbutz Hagoshrim, which means "the bridges," to signify bringing Turkish Jews across from Turkey to Israel, either as visitors to learn about the Holy Land of their Jewish religion, or as permanent settlers.

All around me were landmarks of the fabulous history of ancient Palestine. And there lies the Dan, where arise many of the principal springs that feed the nearby River Jordan, which in turn feeds and links three great lakes: Galilee and Huleh, which were both within sight from the higher hills, and the Dead Sea.

> And the Lord put such a power into the eyes of the Prophet (Moses) that he beheld the whole land from Jordan to the Sea of Galilee, from Mount Hermon to the wilderness. And every place in the land, from the portion of Naphtali to that of Simeon, from that of Reuben to that of Dan.

The water of the River Dan is so icy from its many underground springs that it was almost impossible to swim there, even in the midday heat. All that I could manage was a quick plunge across before one's flesh froze. I walked the kibbutz sheep alongside those icy, flashing waters, and they and I quenched our thirst there when the sun was like a copper cauldron in the white sky of heat pouring down its fire upon us. I walked the sheep also by the lesser rivers of Hazbany, which means "crying waters," and well describes its whirling torrents, and by the quieter, but also swift-flowing, Nhili, which waters the lands of Hagoshrim, going through its center with its music and cool airs. It is not to be wondered at that, on that very site, once stood the palace of an Arab prince.

I write that I "walked" the sheep, but to have the flock accept me as their shepherd and follow where I led them, had not come easily. I took over the shepherd work from Saul, a young Turkish-Jewish poet who had obtained new work as a printer's apprentice outside the kibbutz. He had had many poems published already in Turkey; his poems were not of shepherd life but of the ancient heroes of Turkey. He was now studying Hebrew to be able to write of the Jewish heroes, past and present.

When I arrived at the kibbutz, Saul had only one day remaining before his departure and had taken me at once to meet the sheep which were resting in a field by the River Nhili. There, Succoth-like booths of water-canes had been made to give shade for the flock when the sun was fiercest. The herd was about two hundred, consisting mostly of ewes and a half-dozen rams, including one great king ram with immense curled horns and shaggy hair.

My hours of work were from midday, when I took over the flock as they were resting and sheltering from the sun-heat in the booths, until six in the evening, which was sunset at that time, late summer.

My first day alone with the sheep, as their shepherd, began well. I had merely to watch over them for two hours of rest, then they were to be led out from the shelters to more distant pastures.

The sheep remained quiet in the shade, only troubled by the many kinds of biting flies which preyed on them, causing them to stamp their hooves, and thereby raising clouds of dust. For my part, I sat in the full sun; only my head was protected by a scarf. I basked in the heat, thinking of my coming bathe in the Nhili. I sat alone with the sheep, far from any place and anyone, and happy! If I had possessed a shepherd flute and known how to play it, I would have played a fine tune! As it was, I had only the long shepherd staff with me, which I had taken over from Saul, and it could make little music beyond a drum-like tapping on the sun-baked earth.

When the time came for me to take the sheep to pasture, I wanted to walk them to a nearby fruit garden from which Saul had brought me a capful of delicious crimson and golden pomegranates and purple clusters of small semi-wild grapes. I longed for more of that fruit, and I wanted to see the sheep feeding on the lush herbage which grew in such places, and on the litter of fallen fruits below the trees. Most of the ewes were in-lamb and were in need of ample food to make their unborn lambs strong and healthy.

I walked a few paces from the resting flock and called to them, using the quite ugly cry that the shepherds use in Palestine, and which sounded like a person gargling. I resolved to change this when I knew the sheep better, and to use the old Celtic cattle cry of *"Cusha! Cusha!"* which I had taught to my own goats years ago on the Sussex marshes in England.

Soon I knew that whatever call I made to the flock, it would make no difference, for they were determined not to follow me at all, and intended to remain defiantly huddled together in a great bunch of two hundred animals, in the shade of the sheepfold, for the rest of that day. As calling produced no response I tried prodding some of the sheep on the outside of the flock with my staff, but this also was without effect. I tried forcing my way in amongst the animals, but they closed more tightly together, forming a closely-knitted shawl of gray-white wool, streaked with brown and black in places. Furthermore, the many barbs from the thorny vegetation of Galilee adhered to the wool of the sheep and pricked my limbs even through the long cotton-twill trousers with which the kibbutz had supplied me for my work.

I began to feel desperate. Here I had obtained work which I enjoyed, and a kind home for my dog whilst his broken limb healed – for the Turks loved him – and I would have to abandon the work on the first day. For one cannot be a shepherd if the flock will not follow!

I sat on the ground close to the sheep. I was tearful, also angry with them for spoiling my happiness. If they would have come with me I would have taken good care of them, as I love all sheep.

The dried grasses of summer whispered and sang around me and the reeds slapped their green streaming leafage away in the brook. I thought to myself as I listened to the reeds: "If I pull a strong hollow reed and cut notches in it with a sharp flint, and make some sort of music, the sheep might like me better as their shepherd, and might follow." As a child in England, in the company of my brothers and sisters, we had made reed pipes and played them by the brooks of the pleasant Dales of Derbyshire. So, with some difficulty, I made my pipe and played on it. It made a horrible noise, like wind through a keyhole. And I threw it away.

A ewe came from the flock and approached me and nibbled at the straps of my sandals. She had brown markings on her head and silver patches on her long ears, like silver coins sewn on them. Some other ewes came to the side of the first one and then a young ram also.

I thought next that if I got up from the ground and walked away slowly, a small group might follow me. It would be a beginning; more might come after. I did that; I stroked the ewe with the silver coin-like markings, and she followed at my side. Then the others came – all the flock as I had hoped. They were mine! at least for some months.

I led the sheep flock first towards the grove where Saul had gathered the good fruit. I, too, was able to gather fruit there, although I was rather afraid. Even with the two hundred sheep for company I felt uneasy. To me, the place felt haunted by dispossessed Arabs; most of those deserted Arab gardens, especially in Galilee, seem phantom-possessed. For they are richly fruited and beautiful, and they who planted them and tended them formerly, must have regretted leaving them.

Grapes were few, for it was the end of summer, and the pigeons had cleared most of the golden and purple clusters. But there was a pomegranate feast awaiting the sheep and me. Pomegranates hung in hundreds upon the bushes and trees in their scarlet or green or tawny globes, and the ground was also littered with them. Only pomegranate is a fruit with juice which stains cloth more permanently than most other fruits. I remembered this from Turkey, where the women would take their pomegranates to the Turkish baths; lying naked on the marble slabs of the bath place, they could enjoy the sweet juicy fruits without fear of spoiling their clothes with permanent stains.

I, likewise, took off my shirt and, sitting on the ground in the golden sunlight falling between the trees with the sheep pressing around me, I ate countless pomegranates of both kinds, the mild and sweet ones, and the strong and bitter.

There, surrounding me, were the braided dusks of the crowding vines, and the light coming emerald between the fruit bushes and trees where the sun did not penetrate. There was lush grass also growing in the clearings, and the flock grazed well. They gave to me that good sheep music which I was to come to know so well: mouths pulling at grass and jaws rhythmically champing to the moving hooves. "The golden-hoofed animal," sheep are called, for their eating never destroys vegetation, and their dung and urine fertilize the places where they graze. The warm, good scent of the sheep came to me and I felt love for them, as many other shepherds have loved them.

I thought about the Jewish shepherds who made world history: Moses, David, and Jesus Christ. Christ's tenderness for lambs and sheep, and His knowledge of shepherding them, is evident in many of His parables. Those who do not love animals (except their flesh for eating!) claim that when Christ spoke of sheep He referred only to the human race. I will never accept this. He spoke as a man who loved sheep:

> I am the good shepherd and know my sheep, and am known by them; and I lay down my life for my sheep.

The Talmud tells of Moses and David as shepherds:

> He searches the righteous. How? By judging of the manner in which they attend to the flocks entrusted to their charge.
>
> David, the son of Jesse, He tried in this manner. Before the lambs David set tender grass for food; to the old sheep he gave soft herbs and tender grass, while to the young sheep, able to chew well, he gave old grass, feeding each according to its wants and strength. Therefore the Lord said: 'David, who is able to care for the wants of the flocks entrusted to him, will be able to rule properly over my flock, the people of Israel,' even as it is written, 'After the young flock He brought him to rule over Jacob His people.'
>
> So did the Lord try Moses. While keeping the flock of his father-in-law in the wilderness, a lamb left the flock and ran away. The merciful shepherd pursued it and found it quenching its thirst at a spring by the roadside. 'Poor lamb,' said Moses, 'I did not know that thou wast thirsty,' and after the lamb had finished drinking he took it up tenderly in his arms and carried it back to the flock. Then said God, 'Moses, merciful Moses, if thy love and care is so great for an animal, how much greater will it be exerted for thy fellow-beings; thou shalt lead my people Israel.'

I, too, took the sheep to springs and streams; they are numerous in the hills of Galilee, and always come fresh and cold out of the earth or rock. We drank together and often bathed together, and also ate water-mints and cresses, they and

I, and pulled blackberries from the bushes which bore lush fruits when they grew with their roots in the brooks or rivers.

Only all was not blissful existence with my sheep work. Apart from the biting flies with which the sheep and I had to contend, there were the dust clouds along the lanes, which filled my lungs and almost blinded my eyes, and further, adhering to sweating skin, covered me with filth, so that an evening bath in the River Nihili when my work was ended was an essential. Only water-snakes swam there, lessening the pleasure of my swimming, and there were biting flies awaiting bathers, too!

The rams were quarrelsome. As early as my second day one of the young rams was attacked by the king ram of the flock. The fighting was vicious, the rams rushing at each other with lowered heads, one pounding upon the other in stunning crashes, until I feared that the king ram would kill the young one and then the kibbutz would be angry with me and I would not be allowed to be one of their shepherds. Therefore I took up my long and broad staff, and I myself rushed at the two fighting rams who at that time had their horns locked, the immense curling horns of the king hooking cruelly around the lesser ones of the younger animal.

Taken by surprise, the fighting rams separated, and I then chased off the younger one and the fight was ended. Only the king stood defiantly and gave me such a vicious look that I decided that the animal might well be dangerous and would need watching. Therefore I decided that I should take the trouble to pet him and make him feel friendly towards me. My herbal veterinary work in many lands with all kinds of animals had taught me concerning animal character, and I could usually recognize a bad-hearted one when I met with one.

Accordingly, the following day after the fight between the rams, I kept back crusts of my bread from my midday meal which I always ate in the fields. Some pieces I then fed to the ewe with the silver-coin markings, who was becoming a pet of mine, and was loved by me, and was much at my side, almost taking the place of my dog Fuego when I was away alone with the sheep. The larger portion I took to the king. Piece by piece I fed him with my fingers, meanwhile talking to him in friendliness, for he was handsome to look at, if bad of heart.

Then, when I had fed the last piece of bread to the ram, and he saw that there was no more, he stepped aside from me. With amazing swiftness, considering his great size, he turned and came at me in a rapid charge. My body with protective instinct swung away out of reach of the great horned head. My next instinctive desire was to turn and run away and leave the flock. I wished to do this with my physical body, but my spirit told me to stay. I was still undecided when the ram made a quick return attack. Only this time he had not the advantage of complete surprise, and I hit out at him with my staff and managed a blow on his back. Without that shepherd's staff I would have been helpless and easily overcome by the vicious animal.

I ran next into the midst of the huddled sheep for protection, for I felt sure that the ram would not attack his own kind. I was mistaken; he made two more charges, but he was enraged and did not use his intelligence. Each time I hit him effectively. Fear is more reasonable than anger, and having received three heavy blows from my staff, the king slunk away from me and lost himself, purposely seemingly, amongst the flock. Only, in defeat, his big yellow eyes met mine, and if his expression had been wicked on that day when I had ended his fight with the young ram, on this day it was diabolical! I told myself that during all my time with the flock I would take care that the king ram never again came nearer to me than the distance of my outstretched staff. If he fought at any time with the other rams I would fling my staff at him but would not go near him again, never more would I be within range of his great curled horns.

On my return to the kibbutz that dusk, I asked one of the other shepherds about the king ram. I then learnt that my fears had had good grounds. That ram was of mixed blood, Arab and Israeli, and was a very valuable sire. He had been purchased cheaply from another kibbutz, because he had downed a shepherd there and gouged out one of his eyes. I was shocked that no one had remembered to warn me of the dangerous character of that animal, but also pleased, for I had fought with the animal and defeated him. If I had known of his record, I would have been too afraid to strike him at all, and therefore should fear him more than I did after my successful stand against his attacks. I was thereafter always careful to keep the king ram a good distance from me, but this precaution, that I had to take daily, marred my pleasure in the flock.

The safe return of the two hundred sheep every evening always gave me reason for contentment, for we went to far places and met dangers. Sunset was our time of return. The rose glow of the Galilean sunsets touched the fleeces of the sheep and gave to them increased beauty. A shepherd friend, Eli, one of the first original members of the Turkish kibbutz, and a distant relative of mine, came to meet me most evenings to take over the flock, giving me time to get to my dog and take him to the Nhili, to share my bathing. The cold, swift waters were good massaging for the dog's injured leg.

Often, after the kibbutz evening meal, I would go with my Turkish-Italian friend Ugi to sit in the haystack close by the sheep, which were kept in the court of the former Arab prince's palace. The ruined palace itself was now a storeroom for sheep and cattle food. The warm, sweet scent of the sheep came to us, and many nights we heard the distant howling of the jackal packs. That sound always quickened my heart, being terrible but also exciting. There from the haystack, with eyes half-closed, I would imagine that the sheep sounds were those of the prince's horses and camels, as he came riding home to the waiting women with bells ringing and flutes piping and men's voices singing through those perfect, breathless, starlit nights of Galilee.

Before I left the kibbutz to go to Turkey, a Feast of the Shepherds was held. This was to celebrate the second anniversary of the sheep flock in the kibbutz. It was a new young flock, only the king ram was old. Saul, the former shepherd, whose place I had taken, returned for the celebration. We had several photographs taken, one with him sitting valiantly across the back of the king ram, near me with my pet ewe (see pages 142 and 208).

I did not know what sort of a feast to expect. I hoped that it might be similar to the old Grecian shepherd ones, with the ground or tables spread with ewes' milk cheeses and yogurt and country fruits and garlands of flowers. The festival was to be held in the kibbutz library, so I supposed it would be around a table! It was around a table, but I was only right in that thought, for the rest of the feast was dishes of newly killed and roasted sheep, with bread and wine. Not a flower on the table! Not a fruit! And the countryside was then rich with blossoms of scented oleanders, giant mallows, willow herbs, primrose-tinted purple scabious, and water lilies; there were pomegranates in abundance, apples, pears, oranges and lemons!

My hound had been invited to the gathering and a large bone provided for him. For my part, before I could sit at the table at all, I had to know that the flesh was not that of my pet ewe. I was told that it was from two surplus young rams. Even so, I felt sorry for the rams, and wondered which of the six in the flock had been taken.

I made my feast on bread and wine; my friend Ugi who had been invited to accompany me ate likewise, out of friendship, although he was not a vegetarian.

Toasts were drunk to all shepherds everywhere, and to that ancient craft. Prayers were said for the sheep, that they would have health and fertility, that the ewes would safely bear their lambs, and that all would be protected from the fangs of jackals and foxes, and attacks from eagles and other great birds of prey.

Among the songs sung was an old Hebrew pastoral, telling of the love of a shepherd for a shepherdess in Galilee.

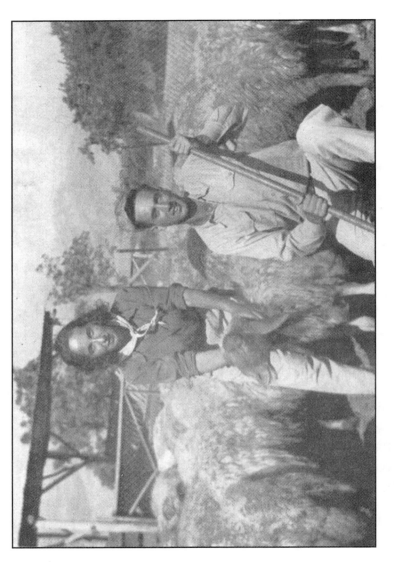

Galilee shepherds: Juliette and Saul

Chapter Ten

Last Days of Summer

Summer is long in Galilee. It moves into autumn without being noticed. Possibly winter comes the same way there, quietly mingling, so that one is uncertain whether autumn has been or winter has come. The winters of Galilee are said to be cold and lifeless; that may be, but the last days of summer are most beautiful, and bring welcome variety in their rains, which freshen the earth and send the quick grass springing up in abundance and the plants to flowering. I particularly remember the rain-lilies, which grew in broad silver lines everywhere around the Lake of Galilee, flowering like the pale rays of the moon.

Those sudden squalls – for which the Lake of Galilee is well known and feared – would give place to driving rain which would last a day or half a day, and turn the streets of Tiberias into places of rushing torrents, quite impossible to cross in some parts, especially by our quarter of Maimoneyeh close below steep hills, where, after the long summertime of baking, the earth could not, at first, absorb the rainwater, which went streaming over it in brown floods.

Those storms at the end of summer caused violent sea-like waves to arise on the lake and brought loud-voiced seagulls to Galilee from the near Acre coast. At such times the waves of the lake were especially perilous, for they then possessed a whirl and a sucking power which dragged bathers to their death. But unlike the true sea, whose waves during and after storms are filled with sand or shingle, the Lake of Galilee waves remained clean, rising in gray-blue and silver heights and flinging foam of absolute whiteness; also they seemed charged with a dynamic power, making it an exciting experience to bathe in those storm waves. My children and I, during those late summer storms, as we bathed in the lake, clung to the shore rocks or to the stumps of the ancient pillars of King Herod's ruined city.

Those old stone columns, as I have written, are to be found in numbers scattered over the southern fields by the Lake of Galilee, and on the hills behind. This granite of Egypt could also be seen crowning Castle Hill above the lake, where once had stood the great palace and temple of Herod. They are made of stone from the quarries of Aswan in Egypt, ancient Seyene. One morning on the deserted lakeshore of summer's ending, my children and I saw history made – or lost – concerning one of those ancient columns; one, like many of them, which had been worn down by time and weather to a mere stump. Only that particular stump was distinguished from all the others that we knew along the stretching lake shore, by having four sculptured scrolls finely modeled around its ground-level base.

We had seen on a previous morning two men probing with iron levers around that particular pillar base. Now it seemed they were back to drag the old stone thing from its bed in the lake shingle where it had rested for nearly two thousand years, and take it away. They were accompanied by a tractor carrying a crane with a steel hawser attached. This hawser, with much difficulty, was fixed in a noose around the old relic, and then all of the power of the two men and a modern machine were exerted to compel the stone thing from its ancient site. For a time it seemed that the relic would resist its removal; that the straining steel hawser would break. We who watched this operation and who loved old things, hoped that would happen and that the men would be compelled to leave the relic where Herod's slaves had set it. But with a sudden sucking noise of water entering a sand-lined vacuum, the big and heavy object was raised and then dragged bumping over the shingle in the direction of the steep bank where the road was.

"They might have wrapped sacking around the scrolls on the column to protect them," I protested to my children, as we watched the slow bumping progress of the old stone being taken away from the lake. The column base measured nearly two feet across its circle and was several feet deep, and, being of granite, was a great weight. But now that it had been lifted out from its protecting and holding shingle bed, it was dragged away with speed.

I called to the men to tell me where they were taking the relic and they said it was going to a museum. I hoped that they meant the museum of Tiberias because it rightly belonged there, but when I questioned them further as to whether this was the case, they pretended not to understand my question and with more speed got the relic up on to the vehicle with the aid of the crane, and then drove away north.

When later I asked the Tiberias museum-keepers if they had the old stone with the scrolls, they did not have it, and were as sorry as we were, my children and I, about its removal. Very possibly it had not gone to a museum at all, but had been sold to someone rich for use as a tea-table! We always felt regret whenever we walked by the water-filled hole where the sculptured column had been for centuries.

As a sign that summer was in its last days, Kubi, the mule-driver, no longer brought his mule Schohorra to bathe in the lake, and we missed their company along the south shore. Jacob, the bus driver, still came to the lake for his sun-bathing and water-bathing, and to eat his luncheon there and read his history books in between driving an Egged

Company bus between Tel Aviv and Tiberias. Only he came less frequently.

Then Itzhak, the gardens-keeper, changed his typical round cotton hat of the Israeli workman, for a hairy cloth cap. He often came to speak with us now that he had more time, for the coming of the rains meant less work for him; his work formerly consisting largely of watering the parched plants and hoeing the earth around them. He favored an individual expression: "Look it!" All of his conversation, in broken Hebrew-English, was interspersed with look it!s in English, with his eyes enlarging behind his bent, tin-rimmed eyeglasses, and his many gold teeth flashing in the sunlight. He had discovered that I was collecting notes for a book on Galilee, and was very regretful that he did not know enough English to be able to help me. "Look it!" he exclaimed. "I no speak English good, if I speak good, look it!, I tell you many things about old Tiberias good for a book." I regretted that he did not know more English, or I more Hebrew, for I am sure he was a very interesting person. As it was, I discovered that he knew much about the ancient Essenes, and also had read most of the writings of the historian Flavius Josephus.

Once, in a violent lake storm, he came like a knight to rescue us. We had our luncheon with us, and I also had my copybook of Galilee notes to which I added lines most days when I saw or learnt more things which seemed of possible interest. I wrote with a fountain pen and all the pages, the ink, the words, six months of daily work, would have been sodden, spoilt, and lost, but for him.

Itzhak hurried us, when the downpour came, to two Jewish houses standing some distance back from the lake, deserted since the Jewish-Arab hostilities because of their lonely position and nearness to the chain of hillside caves. We would never have thought of seeking shelter in the houses.

Once we were in a safe place and the storm could no longer drench us or our possessions, it was exciting to watch the rain deluge, water-carts of it being emptied from the darkened skies. I washed our lettuce, maize, and apples in the rain which splashed down from an old wall. This I usually did in a clean part of the lake, but the storm had come before I had been able to do so. Itzhak would not share our meal with us, apart from having a handful of olives.

"Take care! Take care! He'll break his gold teeth," my children exclaimed to me in English, as the gardens-keeper was heard crunching at the hard olive stones.

Itzhak told us that his own meal was awaiting him, that he ate well, only his daily food took every *pruta* (an Israeli coin) of his wages, which were big wages, but did not pay for more than his meals. He told me: "I work to eat, look it!"

He was one of many who said this in modern Israel. I had not heard that said seven years ago, but then the shops had been nearly empty of any food. Now there was produce in plenty, of all kinds, for purchase, but often there was not enough money to pay the high prices asked. The upkeep of the powerful Israeli Army had to be paid for by the people. As the people were justifiably proud of their army, that burden was accepted; but, even allowing for that expense upon the nation, prices seemed unreasonably high to me, especially in Galilee where the fertile plains yielded an abundance of foods. In families with many children, the wife frequently had to find employment, and even so, there was difficulty in buying sufficient food and clothing.

For my part, I reluctantly sold my camera which had been with me, and served me well, for many years. Only on condition that I could have it back before I left Israel, there yet being many places and things in Galilee which I wanted to photograph. I was planning return visits to the Turkish kibbutz of Hagoshrim, and to the Bedouin village of Toobah, before I departed from Tiberias, which was near to both places, and I wanted to take photographs.

The Bedouins of Toobah are seldom seen in Tiberias now, whereas formerly they had teemed there. I made inquiries concerning this from one of the chiefs of the Tiberias police whom I met on a visit to Mme Avigdor. He told me that all was well with Toobah and that the power of their Sheikh Abou Yussef remained undiminished. It was possible that the Bedouins now shopped in Nazareth, where prices were far cheaper than Tiberias. Whenever I did see Bedouins in Tiberias I bought gifts of sweets for any children who accompanied their parents, and sent messages of goodwill to Abou Yussef and promised that I would be visiting Toobah again before I left Israel. I was awaiting the cooler weather at summer's ending, remembering from before the sweltering heat of the Rosh Pinah plains and hills.

Then one morning I met the Great Lady of Toobah herself, purchasing cloth in Tiberias. Two Bedouin women of her escort were awaiting her outside the shop; another stood at her side within. She herself, in grand manner, was seated at the counter, choosing materials. She was not pregnant as before, but still corpulent, and her amber eyes were as beautiful as ever. I awaited her return into the street. I had not seen her since my journey of apology to Toobah to put right the mistake of a feast prepared and no guests to partake of it.

I greeted the Great Lady as she came out into the sunlight after having made many purchases. I wondered if she would remember me. I had aged much in seven years. Life had been difficult, and I had also had typhus fever when in the Sierra Nevada mountains of southern Spain. I felt that I now looked more like the wrinkled old weaver woman whom I had met at Toobah, than like the girl whom the young Bedouin men had taken on rides across the Rosh Pinah plains, sitting behind them on their swift Arab horses.

However, the Great Lady recognized me instantly, and embraced me. I asked after Abou Yussef and Toobah, and she said that all was well there. She asked me about my hound Fuego, why was he not with me. I told her with intense sadness that he had been killed several years ago when away from me, in New York, hit by a car when he was chasing another hound in the snow. His grave is there on Long Island. Before his death he sired a litter, of which there is a son said to be exactly like him for both beauty and intelligence; he awaits me in America when I can return there.

I told what I could of this to my Bedouin friend, and she sympathized for my loss of Fuego with real feeling in her eyes.

Our conversation was brief because, most of the time I had been speaking with the group of Bedouin women, we had been jostled by passers-by and almost pushed off the pavement into the road. I said nothing, hoping that this was not deliberate action against the Arab women, there being many embittered Nasser refugees from Egypt in Tiberias. I could sympathize with them, as my sister and her French-nationality husband were at that very time refugees from Cairo, living now in France. The fact that my brother-in-law had been royal portrait painter to ex-King Farouk and many later Egyptian princes, had not availed him at all; he had had to leave Egypt.

I especially hoped that the jostling of the Bedouins was not on purpose or general, because a large number of Israelis whom I met, including journalists, took pride in the fair treatment shown to the Arab population in Israel. For the Bible commands the people of Israel: "Love ye therefore the stranger, for ye were strangers in the land of Egypt."

"How do you think we treat the Arabs?" was often asked me with pride by Israeli friends, the questioner feeling that praise was deserved in reply. And there is a Jewish Society which works especially for the fair treatment of the Arab minority. There is also an excellent monthly journal published in Israel, *New Outlook: Middle East Monthly*, which works for friendship between nations in the Middle East, with both Jews and Arabs contributing helpful and topical articles. I highly commend this journal.

I escorted the Bedouin women to the bus for Rosh Pinah and promised to visit their village in the near future. I had a present for Abou Yussef, purchased in the French Camargue, an ornament for wearing on a chain, of a virile black bull, set in a silver filigree pattern looking like the Eastern Star. For the Great Lady of Toobah I had a silver brooch, also of filigree, set with blue stones against the Evil Eye. I looked forward to my visit to Toobah, but awaited cooler traveling days for my young children, and such days seemed as if they would never come.

The late summer brought the graceful long-tailed water wagtails to Galilee. They ran to and fro along the old lake wall by the waterfront, and hopped from rock to rock, sipping from the shoreside pools. The late summer also brought many human immigrants to Israel and to Tiberias. I met with a number of remarkable characters. They came in numbers, not only from Egypt but from the other countries of Arab rulers. The old people from Baghdad brought with them stores of dried flowers and leaves for their medicine and also yogurt cultures in bottles, and wicker baskets for making their milk cheeses. Once, hearing the sound of a drum, I saw what looked like a primitive medicine man passing along the main street of Tiberias and beating a big drum of animal skin stretched over a wooden frame, painted in gaudy colors. The musician was of massive stature and was dressed in a striped pajama suit and plaid cloth bedroom slippers. Such is a common dress amongst oriental people, especially Arabs, who like striped clothing and also comfortable footwear!

The man was followed by a crowd of Tiberias children including many friends of Rafik and Luz, and I let my children join their companions. The man had a dark, round, laughing face, and I think boys and girls would have liked to follow him even if he had not carried the drum with its compelling throbbing music; for, using his hand, he played with much skill. Later I was told that the man with the drum was another Jewish refugee from Egypt and his drum was made from the skin of a lion.

The most memorable Jewish immigrant family whom I met during both of my summers in Galilee, was a family from Kurdistan, recently arrived in Israel by air, and awaiting a bus to take them to a place beyond Safed. All this information was given to me on the air company labels attached to some of their bags and baskets. They had come at the end of summer, but the heat was yet fierce, being one of the very hot and humid days experienced in between the rain storms. The sudden change of air from Kurdistan to that of Tiberias, many hundreds of feet below sea level, seemed to have afflicted the family painfully, and the oldest member was stretched out on the hot pavement amongst the flies and dust, her body heaving with despair, while around her pressed the feet of a typical impatient Israel bus queue.

The most striking of that family from Kurdistan was a dark middle-aged woman, seemingly the mother of the young girl and her two brothers standing near to her. She was unusually tall and towered above the crowd awaiting the same bus. Her powerful body was clothed like a legendary oriental queen's. Apart from her turban-like headdress of sea-green taffeta, not one color of green, but streaked in many shades and shot with blue also, her body was swathed with innumerable lengths of material, wound as tightly as the leafage around a cob of maize. The lengths were entirely unsewn so that she must have been carrying her stocks of material with her in that safe way against theft!

Looking at the materials I felt that their owner had reason to show care for them for they would have brought her a fortune from the dress salons of Paris, London, or New York. Each length was a dream of artistic beauty, if gaudy in some instances. There were velvets, satins, silks and muslins, all heavily embroidered with perfect designs of flowers, foliage, birds, and butterflies, moons and stars. Never in my life have I seen such exquisite colors of materials, nor such shades of embroidery threads, and all applied with remarkable skill.

The swaddling continued down to the tops of the wearer's purple velvet slippers, fitted with golden buckles in the form of crescent moons. Her eyes and her abundant loose-hanging hair were badger-black, her face like old copperware, dark and glowing, with the nose Semitic-form and powerful, with wide nostrils. She wore a crowd of bangles reaching high up her thick forearms which were not covered by the materials. Some of the bangles were plain gold and silver, others were of those metals but finely worked, some were of tortoiseshell, ebony, and lapis lazuli. But most unforgettable of all was an object which she held carefully in her right hand: a teapot!

Oh, that teapot! That such a perfect thing could be made by man in this world! No writing can describe beauty of that degree; the texture of its porcelain, lustrous as Persian or Mexican pearls, the porcelain inset with encircling bands of gold, and decorated with the forms of blood-red roses on a sulfur yellow background. Those exquisite red roses were in all stages of growth, from youngest budding to the most fully opened flower, casting petals. In the center of the teapot lid was set a large ruby stone. It could not have been a real stone, or its value would have provided a more comfortable form of travel than an Israeli bus.

Thinking of the approaching bus travel, I feared for the safety of that precious teapot, its fragile spout which arched like the neck of a golden swan – if there are golden swans – and the equally fragile handle. Surely such a rare object should have been carried carefully in a basket, surrounded with protective paddings. I was considering, for the sake of art in the world, of hastening to a shop and purchasing basket and straw to present to the owner of the teapot for its safety, when my intention was thwarted by the arrival of the bus. I was, however, able to stand by the immigrants from Kurdistan and give warning cries of "Take care of that teapot!" to the other jostling passengers; and owner and pot were helped into the bus to the safety of a corner seat.

The rest of the family then also had to be aided into the bus, as they seemed afraid of it. Each one of them was remarkable. The children went first, the girl slender, judging from her wrists and ankles, for like her mother she was carrying on her person many lengths of magnificent cloths, and it was difficult to make out the shape of her figure. She wore bracelets around her ankles, broad bands of old, dull silver, with a big, wrought-silver rose attached to each one. The boys wore velvet turbans of Indian rajah style, one of ruby velvet, the other of jade. One wore a fine white silken shirt with flowing sleeves, and baggy trousers of a dull red cloth, the other a vulgar South Sea Islands cotton beach shirt, and the same type of baggy red trousers as his brother. All three children were dark-skinned like their mother, and of straight, proud carriage, with fine-featured faces. "Well-bred" could rightly be applied to them.

The father was of such short and squat stature that he looked an absurd mate for the towering woman with her teapot; the top of his head barely reached to the woman's waist. Only it was difficult to judge the man's height on account of his large black turban, shot with golden thread, made of taffeta similar to the headdress which his wife wore. In the center of the forehead part of the turban was a gold brooch of oval shape, set with pearls. His jacket was of black-flannel type cloth and his trousers, ordinary of cut, were of white flannel striped with black.

Finally the old woman of their family had got on to her feet when the bus was almost ready to depart, taking with her, on her fine gown of peacock-patterned silk, much debris from the pavement: dust, sunflower seed castings, melon pips, toffee papers, and used bus tickets, all adhering to the sweat-damped material.

I was pleased to see the whole family safely on the bus, for the woman sprawling on the pavement had nearly been stepped upon many times by the ruthless feet of the bus queues. "Too few buses for the rapidly increasing population," I was told in explanation of the always unpleasant experience of these queues. Also it was said that a large proportion of the people in the queues had been in Nazi concentration camps and that they were alive and living in freedom today in Israel and elsewhere because they had ruthlessly fought for their survival; and in the bus queues they were still instinctively fighting as before. I argued back that I am sure that many of the concentration camp victims survived differently, through the hand of God reaching down to save them. Somewhere in the Bible there is such a promise: two will be sleeping in one bed and one will be taken.

Numerous people in modern Israel have concentration camp numbers branded on their arms, and on seeing them, I always thought of gas chambers, Hitler, tortures, and how these branded numbers must evoke in their possessors – whenever their eyes caught sight of them in daily life – such horror, and how wonderful it is that those persons now lived in freedom in a Jewish state which had outlived Hitler. Memorial trees are planted on the hill slopes of Israel, creating new forests in memory of the Jews whom Hitler murdered; one tree for each Nazi victim is aimed at. That will mean millions and millions of trees, for Hitler's victims were not confined to Europe alone; Yugoslavia, Bulgaria, Greece, even as far as the Island of Roses – all lost their teeming multitudes of Jews to Hitler and his gas chambers. And I have seen concentration camp numbers on people from all these countries, and from many others. The miraculous survival of the Tunisian Jews is said to be due to the absolute refusal of the old Bey of Tunis to allow any of his people – and he included the Jews as his people – to be killed in this terrible way. There are signs of gas chamber sites in Tunisia, but work on them was never completed.

When I commented on the lack of manners in queues and elsewhere in Israel, I was told that in twenty years' time there will be good manners. At present it is a question of the survival of a young country and there were more important things to take the attention of the State than manners. In the days of the "Wild West" of America there had been no time for good manners. I wondered about this; and meanwhile I was glad to see the Kurdistan family safely on the crowded bus. Other Tiberias travelers, known to me, who were going beyond the destination of that family, promised me they would help the new immigrants off the bus, together with their baggage, and the teapot.

After the rains, with the lessening of the heat and the dust, my children and I were able to travel to new places in Galilee, or close to its borders. As I have written, all over Galilee are places of great beauty or historic interest; often the two are combined.

It was during our last days that we visited the piece of waste land opposite the north shore of the Lake of Galilee, where the Tiberias boys play football. An area has been fenced off for excavations, as underground dwellings have been found there of similar type to those occupied by the family of the Virgin Mary, and the Holy Family, and others of Nazareth. These dwellings possess the same underground passages, deep rainwater cisterns and pipes, and several have big stone communal family eating bowls.

Summer in Galilee

In the Galil, in the region of Tiberias, the tombs of pre-historic cave dwellers of the early Stone Age have been found, dating from 2.7 million ago to 200,000 years ago. Therefore the area is very old in the history of man.

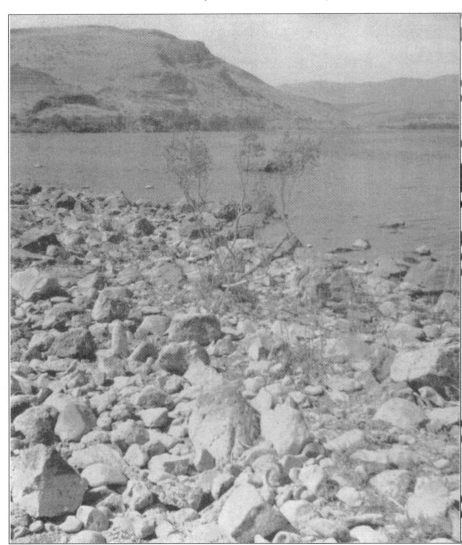

View across Lake Galilee toward Mary's Pool

We at last found the weather cool enough to walk along the hot open road to the village of Magdala, or Migdal, with its splendid fig trees. There can be no doubt that Mary, surnamed Magdalene, received her name from there. The coast around that village, on the north shore of the Lake of Galilee, has a tragic history. Again and again the Galileans of that area, known for their valiant and passionate character, rose against the Romans, always to be subdued and driven into the very lake, to die there in baths of blood.

Farther back towards Tiberias, a short distance from Magdala, are the Russian gardens. Here there are cold and warm springs of water. The Russians – believing this site to be the birthplace of Mary Magdalene, and certainly to be the warm spring-fed pool where she bathed – settled there after the World War; the place since has become holy ground.

There are lovely places in the world; this pool of Mary Magdalene by the shore of the Lake of Galilee, is one of them. It is of the ring – Galil – shape, and its base is of a peculiar blue-gray shingle, showing clearly through the shining, limpid water which covers it deeply. And all the while through this water the warm spring bubbles up, like whirling silver smoke rising up to the surface of the pool, that endless rise and then outward dispersal of the warm water.

There is some shade given over Mary's pool, a blessing in that summer climate of the great heat; the overhanging crags give shade, and also a eucalyptus tree. The black and white ice birds were diving from this tree to spear small fish in the pool, and kingfishers veered up from the rocks as we drew near to the place. It was certainly a place of birds also, and further of butterflies; the Great and the Little Ladies of the Lake species, with their wings of orange and white, were there in numbers.

Then over the craggy heights above the water there hung in cascades of snow, small, white veronica-type flowers of pungent honey scent, singing with the crowding bees. I have not found a similar rock-flower in any other part of Galilee. To that quiet and perfect place, quite lonely in its distance from Magdala, and far from Tiberias, Mary Magdalene used to come to bathe.

Now a small chapel and a Young Men's Christian Association hostel stand near by; that is all. The place was very quiet when we were there, for it was an unseasonable time of the year for visitors to Galilee. It was so quiet there that my children and I thought we could hear the wing sounds of the ice birds as they spread wings for their fish-questing plunge into Mary's pool.

Close by, facing the Christian hostel, we could see the site of Rakath. Barren rocks, resembling ruins, show where Joshua, the son of Nun, destroyed a city and laid a curse upon the place that it should never be inhabited. Only families of ravens defy Joshua's curse.

We traveled to the former Canaanite town and old seaport of Acre, standing in its burning plain on the border of Galilee, with its medieval atmosphere and, for me, especially, the spirit of the Crusaders everywhere. The Crusaders had made Acre their chief port in the Holy Land; the old fortress of the Knights Hospitaller still stands. But it is the beautiful mosque of Acre which dominates the scene, as it rests like a silver tulip bulb over the crowding white houses still largely populated by Arabs. Whilst we were there, the leaves of the grape vines, turned golden and silver at summer's end, drifted across the town like flights of butterflies and settled upon our sandaled feet.

I bought the delicious and special bread of Acre for us to eat as we explored the old bazaars. The bread is sold in the early morning, warm from the ovens. It comes in round, flat cobs, which the bread sellers split open and sprinkle heavily with the delicious pungent powdered herbs collectively called *Zahtar*, which we had also had in Nazareth, but which never tasted better than when supplied with the bread of Acre.

In the bazaars we bought oriental necklaces made from wooden beads and some gaudy, but warm, head-scarves for our sea journey soon forthcoming. Only before we left Galilee and Israel for Paris, we had two sentimental journeys to make: to the Turkish kibbutz of Hagoshrim in Upper Galilee, where I had worked as a shepherd and known my happiest months of all my time spent in Galilee, and also to visit the Bedouin village of Toobah, also in Upper Galilee but not so far north as Hagoshrim.

We went in early September to the Turkish kibbutz. It was no longer Turkish, I had been told, for the Turks had joined with another older kibbutz whose members were mostly Hungarian. Also the Emir's palace had been restored in part and was now a prosperous, if small, guest house, where many of the chiefs of the Israeli Government went to rest.

The whole journey back up into the hills of Galilee was a revelation for me: for there from the time that we left Rosh Pinah to go to the lands of Hagoshrim, the extraordinary progress made by the Israeli people since I had last passed that way was set out before my eyes. I could see below me the drained lands reclaimed from the former swamps of Huleh, and along the winding mountain road former tracts of wilderness had become villages. There was even an entirely new town, with the name of Kiryat Shmona, possessing school, hospital, post office, and numerous shops and houses, also having a large and busy motor-bus station and center. Yet I found Hagoshrim the greatest revelation of all.

Where before there had once been a collection of shacks with the exception of the good new library, set by the flashing waters of the River Nhili, there was now by the same river a further Galilean village! In addition to the restored part of the ruined palace building, there were now a hundred or more villa-type houses set in flowering gardens, the rose bushes being especially notable, and the green lawns; with so much sweet water, lawns were no great difficulty.

Large play lawns had been made for the children. There were the communal nurseries and dormitories of the typical kibbutz life; there was a vast new dining hall and big kitchens for preparing and cooking the meals served there. Now good and varied meals were served; on my previous visit, in those pioneer years of hardship, our diet had been mainly dry bread, potatoes, olives, soup, and artificial white cheese, with margarine considered a luxury when it was available. Fruit had been almost unknown and I remembered how I had blessed my shepherd work because it had given me access to the deserted Arab fruit gardens. Now the kibbutz boasted far-stretching melon fields and apple orchards.

The new cattle buildings were magnificent and my Turkish friend, Sara from Smyrna, had helped to build up a splendid herd. Unfortunately, there were many battery houses for the poultry. I hate these cruel battery houses in whatever country I see them, and I see them almost everywhere. Never have animals been so exploited as today; the battery houses are but one example.

There were extensive fish ponds now for the breeding of carp. Before there had been three small ponds; now there were acres under water, and in such cold healthful water the fish were flourishing. With such fertile land and an abundance of water, the kibbutz only lacked a sufficiency of workers to make it an earthly paradise, in the opinion of the experts. I agreed with them, but hoped the mice would be banished from Hagoshrim in time, for there should be no mice in paradise! I know of no lovelier part of Israel, when one gets away from the crowding new people, there in the quiet places with waters singing and the hill breezes stirring the grasses, reeds, and waterside flowers.

I know a small circular pool away from the River Nhili,

fed by springs, where it is a delight to bathe. It has much the look of Mary Magdalene's pool by the Lake of Galilee, but whereas there the water is warmed by the hot spring which rises near the front of that pool, the one beyond Hagoshrim is formed from springs which seem to be of melted snow, so cold they flow. Giant mallows are reflected there, as the springs flow slow, and also the golden hedges of giant St. John's wort, as high as twenty feet, and the ostrich-like plumes of the flowering water-canes give out a sweet, heavy scent. Canes and maize growing in masses emit a rich perfume at flowering time.

Another memorable place for water and plants was the restored gardens of the former Emir's palace. Under a wilderness of nettles, thistles, and thorns, such as rapidly possess untended land in Israel, acres of old terraced gardens – with streambeds through which water of the Nhili and other springs had once coursed – were discovered and restored, with the waters diverted to flow there again. The same aromatic rosemary, myrtle, and altabacca plants grew in their former places, crowding on the walls above the streams. Figs dropped, golden and black, into the water, pomegranates ripened their fruit of fire without and cool honey within, and bananas grew in their rich green groves. In the many trees giving fruits and shade, sweet-voiced turtledoves could be heard, supposed to be moaning because love is inconstant; they know, and mourn therefore.

My children and I ran, enchanted, from terrace to terrace, and then pulled and ate handfuls of pungent watercress as we bathed in the cool brooks of those gardens.

Seven years would be sure to have brought many changes amongst my former friends in the kibbutz, and especially in such a changing country as Israel. Most of my friends had left the kibbutz, all the shepherds had gone with the exception of my relative Eli, also of Smyrna, who was now a teacher of languages to the kibbutz children, and the young Jewish students who come every year to the kibbutzim of Israel to work on the land and to learn Hebrew. And the sheep had gone with the shepherds! How sad that was. For Hagoshrim is natural sheep and goat land, with endless abundant grazing for those animals, and sweet water for their drinking, and therefore wonderful stock and herds could be established in such a territory. I was told that when the original shepherds left, the other kibbutz members found the work too monotonous, and none could be found to shepherd the sheep. (And what of my pet ewe with the silver-coin markings on her ears! No one could tell me what had become of her.) Shepherd work monotonous! Every hour of it had been pleasure for me. Cleaning out the dirty cages of the hen battery houses — that is both boring and disgusting work! — yet poultry had replaced the sheep.

My Turko-Italian friend Ugi had left the kibbutz for which he had worked so hard, and had married, and like myself had two children. I went alone one night to visit again the place by the old sheep byres, where the big haystacks had been in the Emir's palace court, and where Ugi and I had liked to spend our evenings after the communal meal. Of all the men who have been my friends, he was the kindest to me. He was a philosopher and had compelled me to alter my character; therefore he can never be forgotten.

It was a Japanese poet who wrote:

> These meetings in dreams
> How sad they are!
> When, waking up startled
> One gropes about—
> And there is no contact to the hand. (Manyo Shu ca.704 C.E.)

My hound Fuego used to be in the court with us also, and he had gone forever, apart from living on, to some extent, in the Afghans which he had sired in America.

How hard we had all worked seven years ago to provide the food needed urgently for the crowding immigrants. My shepherd task had never been hard, but Ugi had driven a tractor for endless hours on open fields, through clouds of dust beneath a fierce sun. There had been the other hard work for me before coming to Hagoshrim. That work, especially in the old-type kibbutzim, had been slavish, often. I remember an American immigrant, David, an M.A. with literary honors, who used to work alongside me and chant lines from Alice in Wonderland, concerning Old Father William, as, heads almost touching the ground, we planted tomato seedlings, or gathered cucumbers, or low-growing sweet peppers, toiling with twenty young men and women – or more. The verse ended appropriately for us:

> 'You are old Father William,' the young man said,
> 'And have grown most uncommonly fat,
> And yet you incessantly stand on your head,
> Pray what is the reason of that!'

When the work grew truly bitter, such as lifting and sacking acres of potatoes behind a potato-harvesting machine, many workers would sing the mournful chant of the concentration camps, which it is said the Jews would take up and chant on their way to the gas chambers: "My Hope."

> Ani ma-amin, ani ma-amin, ani ma-amin,
> B'viat hamashiach.
> B'viat hamashiach, ani ma-amin.

I also remember the singing of the Yemenite men as they passed by every evening returning to the big camps in which the Yemenites were usually housed in those days. They went by always in single file, carrying their kettles and cooking pots, for, being very orthodox in religion, they wanted to make sure that milk pots or plates were not mixed with those for meat or vice versa, and to ensure this, they usually prepared their own food over brushwood fires. Their song was mournful and haunting, and – as their work on the kibbutz when I was there was mostly stone clearance from the fields – I felt that they sang unknowingly a dirge for the Israeli earth. For I feel that it is wrong to move stones in such endless quantities to enable rapid tractor cultivation. The stones in land such as Palestine's – where there is little more than a few inches of fertile top-soil and the rest is sand or shale – effectively and permanently hold down the surface soil against erosion; further they conserve moisture, especially those famous dews of Israel, and regulate the temperature of the earth, absorbing the heat by day to keep the soil from becoming over-baked, and giving out the heat by night to prevent over-chilling; all this I observed for myself

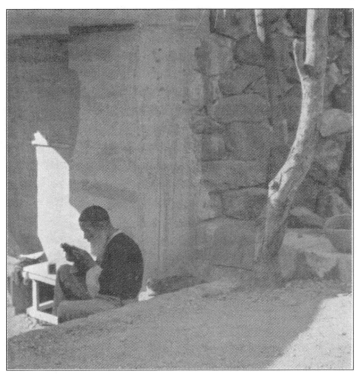

Prayer in the holy city of Tiberias

as a field worker. But many agriculturists far better able to know the facts of soil care than myself, hold this opinion and consider that only obstacle rocks, not the stones, should be removed from the fields.

I believe that primitive agricultural method of scratching the earth surface with hand-tools, is right, is better for the present and future life of the soil, and grows far better-tasting and more healthful crops. Because I admire Hagoshrim and have spent many happy months there, I have sent already many – and shall send more – books on natural farming methods, as I would loathe to see those fertile lands of Hagoshrim rendered so barren by unnatural high-speed modern agriculture that crops could not be grown at all without heavy use of artificial chemical fertilizers, as was the case in several old kibbutzim which I saw, many with their crops diseased.

It is of special interest that Lady Eve Balfour, daughter of the great statesman, Earl Balfour, who helped to restore Palestine to the Jewish nation, is one of the leaders of a powerful English agricultural movement, "The Soil Association."

I am very pleased that at Amrim, near the Acre-Safed highway, a vegetarian village has been set up similar to the ancient Essene settlements, and Amrim's main object will be to farm by natural organic methods. Another similar settlement is planned for Magdala; I would like to visit there.

One of the most impressive things about Hagoshrim, and for most of Upper Galilee, was the disappearance of the mosquitoes. Formerly at every dusk they had come up from the nearby swamp into which Huleh Lake spread itself, in literally ravenous, hissing clouds. Certainly there were still mosquitoes about on the lands of Hagoshrim by night, with so much artificial water there (the fish ponds), but the former menacing clouds had gone; man and beast were freed from their nightly affliction, and it was a great Israeli achievement which I am glad to have witnessed.

I had left my other sentimental journey, the return to Abou Yussef's Toobah, until literally my last days. My children and I had already left Tiberias and were staying in a Haifa hotel close by the port from where we were sailing the next day, after the planned Toobah visit. I had delayed so long because my camera had not been returned to me to take photographs; it was, however, promised faithfully for this last day, and I was going to leave my passport, at my own suggestion, with the camera owner while I had the use of it again. I was to break my journey in Tiberias, on the way to Rosh Pinah, and there collect my camera and be joined by an Arabic-speaking woman friend who was to be an escort to Toobah.

That journey began badly. Summer was positively over; we were into November, but the sun shone down with summertime fierceness from the early morning hours. The journey from Haifa to Tiberias was stifling and I doubted if I would ever get my young children across the burning plains beyond Rosh Pinah up to Toobah. The three-year-old Luz was not yet hardened to fierce heat as were Rafik and I. Then, on arrival in Tiberias I found that my camera was still not forthcoming. Finally, when I had raged for half an hour, I was taken across to a camera shop and there loaned one of the same make as my own, into which I put one of my last two fine films which I had carefully kept for final photographs. Maybe it was the same make, but it felt like a piece of tin in my hands compared with my former camera which had served me well for many years. Even though that one had not been a first-class camera, its lens had given photographs clear enough for reproduction, and that had sufficed. The one now lent to me was the best available, but as I examined it I knew it was trash, and not worth the work which always has to go into taking photographs of any merit at all.

And I had waited so patiently for my camera! I had even dreamed about it while in the Haifa hotel – dreamed that I was standing on my head like Old Father William and taking pictures that way! There were many yet that I had planned to take for this, my future Galilee book: the rain lilies massed around the tottering pillars of the ruins of King Herod's city; the Lake of Galilee seen through the mesh of drying fishing-nets; the excavations on the Tiberias football field, including the big stone family eating bowl; camels; and above all, Toobah! those black 'tents of Kedar,' the black-and-tan goats; and then, with much care, Abou Yussef and his people.

I had already written to inform Abou Yussef that I was bringing a good camera with me on my visit and hoped to take better pictures this time. Then, also, I had written him to remember all the trouble of my last visit, and he must know that circumstances beyond my control might prevent my arrival. If I was not at Toobah before two o'clock of the afternoon, I said, I would not reach there. Therefore I now sent him my small gift of a black Spanish bull, said to represent strength and courage, symbolic to me of the Bedouins of Toobah. If I did not come to his village this year he could be sure that I would come some later time.

That was a pessimistic way to start a sentimental journey, but it was soon shown to me that I had been right to nourish such forebodings. Not only was my camera not in Tiberias for me, but further my Arabic-speaking escort had left a message of apology that her husband would not let her go to Toobah! Why did so many persons fear that place which for me was in all ways wonderful! Well, I decided, my two children could be my escorts.

We arrived at Rosh Pinah to find what I had feared when I saw what type of morning had dawned. The plains beyond the bus station shimmered with heat. Good enough for me, I loved such heat, but it would be a toilsome walk for two young children, and our water flask was small.

We set off across the golden plains, golden with midday sunlight and also the color of the earth heat-baked to ochre. Despite the parched state of the ground, wherever there were surface dips or hollows for morning dew to gather, autumn crocuses had come forth in their cups of palest purple, like the Morning Star. And there were finger-high blue scillas of sweet scent. Those unexpected flowers lured Rafik and Luz onwards, as wild flowers have lured children since they were both on earth.

The young boy and girl walked onwards valiantly; they had long learnt to pace quickly at my side; only they soon drank up all the water that I carried. Foolishly I had told them that our water supply was very limited until we got to Toobah. Both children then began to satisfy an urgent thirst, one against the other, until soon there was not a drop of water left. Shortly I knew there would come more insistent demands for "Water! Water! Give us water!" as the Crusaders cried when in the Holy Land as they had fought with the Saracens out on the burning plains, especially in the environs of Galilee; but, as with the Crusaders, there was no more water to be had. Rafik had brought his rosewood flute with him, and I told him to pipe on this to help us along.

Soon the children carried bunches of the autumn crocuses and sweet scillas and I decided to photograph them with their flowers of Galilee. We had found colorful feathers dropped by pigeons and other birds, including some bright blue ones, and put them in our headscarves. Rafik wore one of the round, cotton Israeli hats and I tucked his flowers and feathers in the hatband. I decided to take my first photograph of the new film. But, as I have said, the camera loaned to me in place of my former one, felt like a piece of tin in my hand. There was not, I found on careful examination, even speed control or range-finder available on it. I decided that I could not possibly take such an inferior camera with me to photograph the people of Toobah. Better to have no camera with me at all! I took one miserable photograph of Rafik and Luz and then found a hiding place for the thing beneath a thorn bush, where I arranged handfuls of dry grass for further concealment of the rejected camera. I could collect it on the return walk. I made careful note of the exact position of the concealing thorn bush.

The children and I walked onwards for another half-hour or more. The midday hours had long passed, yet the heat of the sun had diminished little. *"Mayim karim! Mayim karim!"* (cold water) came the whine in Hebrew from my children.

We mounted the brow of a hill to descend again to the onwards-stretching plain, when I saw something wonderful – not the black tents of Kedar alas, but the square houses of Abou Yussef and the family Abdullah.

"Toobah! Toobah! Come and see Toobah!" I called to my children, who had lagged behind.

They mounted the hill eagerly to my side. "Where are the black tents?" Rafik asked.

"They are farther back. The houses can be seen because they are built on the hill ridge and are taller."

"It's the black tents I want to see!" the boy protested obstinately.

"But that must be Abou Yussef's house – that middle one – and there to the left is the House of Abdullah! I've told you about these. Surely you are interested?"

"We want to see the black tents, Mama," both children told me, almost tearfully.

And how far away Toobah looked yet – the houses barely visible against the shimmering sky. Then we saw something else, a big lorry mounting a distant road towards Toobah, and coming from the direction of Rosh Pinah. (Later I was told that the lorry had been sent to look for us and convey us to Toobah.) I felt with despair that that lorry was on the right road for Toobah from Rosh Pinah, and I was taking my children along a wrong one. I had been making for the small Arab cemetery, from where the road mounted to Toobah. But except for riding towards there several times on the back of the Toobah men's horses I had never before gone to the Bedouin village from Rosh Pinah; always from the kibbutz lands. I saw plainly that the journey to Toobah this time was hopeless. In later years the children would be riding ponies and I could take them easily to Toobah that way.

"We'll have to turn back," I informed Rafik and Luz. "Toobah is too far away. I'll never get you there and back again. We'll go another year and I'll hire ponies for you."

Both children loved to ride things, only as yet their steeds had been nothing more ambitious than wooden horses of fairgrounds and an occasional journey on donkey-back. Rafik and Luz had been looking forward to Toobah for many weeks, but both now accepted my decision without protest. Thirst makes an unpleasant companion on any road, and had been our companion overlong on this excursion.

'Look!' Luz suddenly called to us. "There are flying roses!' She indicated a sight of beauty. Over the ridge of the hillock on which we then stood, came a flight of brown crickets, only the inner parts of their wings were of a rose-pink color. Both children called out in delight as the crickets came past us, skimming over the autumn crocuses which pressed against our feet.

"They are insects," Rafik confirmed.

"They are crickets with rose-wings," I told them further. At least we saw much beauty on that walk towards Toobah. Not only the wild flowers, but many kinds of birds, from several species of pigeons, including turtledoves of the bronze plumage, to the brilliant king birds of the Jordan Valley.

The decision made, I was not over-disappointed. I felt I was looking very unattractive – over-thin, my clothes now

ill-fitting on my body. High prices of food had made meals
too small for me many times during our long stay in Galilee.
Indeed, the only time that we had really feasted had been
during the two weeks at the Turkish kibbutz, when the food
given to us had looked like mountains compared with the
usual molehills of our rations that I had been able to afford!

"We look so tired and dusty," I apologized, "and I have
changed too much. I did not look like this before, when they
knew me at Toobah!"

"You look very old," Rafik said. He knew what to say;
he had heard that cry from me so many times, as I stood
before a mirror.

"Yes," I agreed. "I look very old. Now let us turn our backs
on the sun and run as far as we can away to Rosh Pinah."

The three of us waved our hands to Toobah and began
to run. "I shall take you there a better year," I promised.
"We might have our Afghan hound, Fuego's son, with us by
then. Come now, run! I shall buy lemons at Rosh Pinah,
and will crush them into our drinks of water, and you can
eat more of the sugar almonds I have with me for the Toobah
children."

The children contested with each other as to how many
glasses of lemon water they would enjoy at our journey's
ending.

We reached Rosh Pinah before the late noon. It had
been quicker returning than going, with our backs now to
the sun and no climb ahead of us.

At the Egged bus station one of the staff could speak
English, and moreover was friendly toward the Toobah
Arabs. I remembered him from before. I left the brooch for
the Great Lady of Toobah with him, and then asking for a
sheet of paper, wrote a message of explanation to Abou
Yussef, telling him that we had got half-way to Toobah this
time, but would get the whole way there on my next visit to
Galilee.

The Egged man promised to translate this into Arabic when the Toobah people called there on the morrow. He would tell them that he had seen the children and me. He said also that I could not possibly have got young children on foot to Toobah in the heat of the day. It was a two hours' brisk walk or more from Rosh Pinah even for an adult.

We had time on our hands before our return to Haifa; therefore I decided to leave the bus as it approached the north shore of the Lake of Galilee. We could then bathe away the dust of our long walk and return slowly on foot to Tiberias in the cool of the evening, leave the camera there, and take a late bus back to Haifa, which meant that we would be passing through Nazareth in full moonlight, as I loved to see that holy city.

On our way back to Tiberias we would be able to visit our friend Shimon, who was the watchman for a new landing-stage for fishing boats which was being built out into the lake by a work party of Hungarian immigrants. Shimon was one of our last friends that we made in Israel, and amongst the few whom we liked best. He belonged to the last days of summer. We had met him then and watched summer's ending with him, the leaves falling from the trees and the seagulls arriving on the lake to feast on the wrack from the many storms. We bathed in a secluded willow-screened place and watched the sun setting over the water, and stayed until the bats came. Rafik and Luz feasted on the sugar almonds of many colors which I had purchased in quantities for the Toobah children. Those almonds had helped to allay their disappointment that they were leaving Galilee without having seen the black tents of the Bedouins.

All the way along the lake road to the green caravan of Shimon the watchman, we talked about Galilee: Do you remember this and that? Do you remember?

Fragments of cloud accompanied us across the sky above, as we walked. The fragments were colored coral, orange, and flame, and we decided that they were the fire-birds of ancient oriental myth, birds of the crested heads and streaming tails, and with drooping plumes such as are worn also by birds of paradise. We left the fire-birds behind when we came to Shimon's caravan and entered the cool, shady interior.

The watchman was there, young and handsome, of old Jewish Palestinian stock, his hair dark and wiry, growing in long side pieces, and he had a wide black moustache. His skin was bronzed like his brass coffee pot. My children greeted him with affection, and we told him that it was our farewell visit.

"Ah! Julia! Stay in Israel with your children," he said. "You'll find no better land."

Rafik asked Shimon to play his mouth-organ; he would play his flute. We had that music then, beautiful Hebrew tunes from the man, and noise from the boy. We shared out the last of the sugar almonds.

We stayed until the moon rose over the lake: always a sight of splendor, the turning of those wide waters into a luminous wash of silver. We could see this from the back window of the caravan: its door faced the road.

Shimon repeated many times between his bittersweet tunes: "Ah, Julia, stay in Israel."

But I knew that that was not the proper time for us to stay on in Israel, despite all the interest and beauty of Galilee, and our love for its lake. My work was yet elsewhere.

Only I knew surely I had not seen my last summer in Galilee. There would be other summers to come, God willing.

The pigeons of Galilee are homing over the lake; loud in the hot, windless, evening, is heard the tumult of their quick wings. They travel the twilit sky with the circumstance of an army: the evening stars are their lights. The nervous foliage of the eucalyptus trees trembles as the teeming birds surge over them — whispering eucalyptus leaves.

Summer in Galilee

In all colors of plumage they are seen, the pigeons of Galilee: lily-white and silver, and the gray-green of the olive groves, bronze of pomegranate or the near black of old basalt stones. As their feathers are iridescent, these birds are multi-tinted, especially their breasts and heads, and shimmer in the purple Galilean dusk, as painted they are as the famed wild anemones of the Holy Land which in springtime swaddle the foothills around the lake with striped cloths of oriental brilliance.

All are colored except the white doves amongst the pigeons, which are merely touched with silver light like rain lilies now flowering.

Homewards the pigeons fly to the rocky places and deep caves of the hills by the lake. Also to the ruins of Crusader forts, to ancient palaces, temples, churches and mosques, where Galilean history has been made, which is eternal.

The End

Copyright Notice

Acknowledgments

For the current edition, © 2011

A Gypsy wink and a big basket of thanks to the wise women who made this book a reality:

- **Jane Bond** and **Kimberly Eve** for turning Juliette's words into electrons.
- **Kimberly Eve** for her wonderful cover illustrations, interior illustrations and design skills.
- **Jennifer Jo Stevens** for seeing to the never-ending details: the quotes, the numbers, the codes, the facts.
- **Betsy Grace Sandlin**, best friend of words and guardian of the commas.
- **Rose Weissman**, for diligent, delightful assistance.
- **Rev. Ursula Carrie Wilkerson** for scanning photos.
- **Andrea Dworkin** for design assistance.
- **Susun Weed**, for typesetting, editing, designing, and keeping it all humming along.
- Our **guardians**, **grandmothers**, **spirit sisters**, and the **Ancient Ones**.

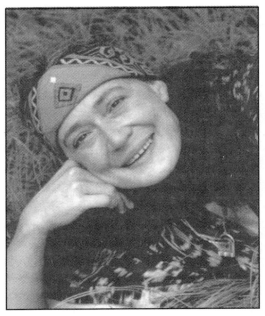

Susun S. Weed (left), editor-in-chief of Ash Tree Publishing, shamanic herbalist, goatkeeper, and lover of women, is thrilled to have this chance to bring Juliette's words and wisdom to the current generation of herbalists.

Kimberly Eve (right) is head of the art department and chief artist at Ash Tree Publishing. She has worked to bring several of Juliette's books back into print.

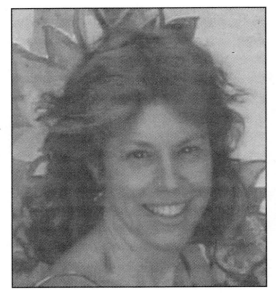

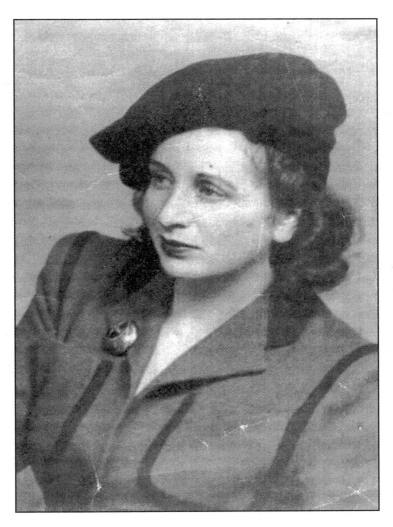

**Juliette de Bairacli Levy** (1911–2009) is honored as the grandmother of modern American herbalism. She has devoted her life to the health and well being of domesticated animals, especially dogs. Her herbals and memoirs have been in print, and in use, for over fifty years.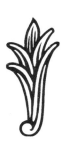

Herbal Index

Other books you will want to read from

Ash Tree Publishing
Women's Health, Women's Spirituality

Wise Woman Herbal Series
best-sellers by
Susun S Weed

Wise Woman Herbal for the Childbearing Year $11.95
Healing Wise, Everyone's Herbal $17.95
New Menopausal Years, The Wise Woman Way $16.95
Breast Cancer? Breast Health! The Wise Woman Way $21.95
Down There, The Wise Woman Way $29.95

Herbals of Our Foremothers Series
classics by
Juliette de Bairacli Levy

Nature's Children $11.95
Common Herbs for Natural Health $11.95
Traveler's Joy $11.95
Spanish Mountain Life $16.95
Summer in Galilee $24.95
A Gypsy in New York $21.95

and, by **Maida Silverman**
A City Herbal $13.95

To order:
- Visit www.wisewomanbookshop.com
- Write to PO Box 64, Woodstock, NY 12498

Prices subject to change.

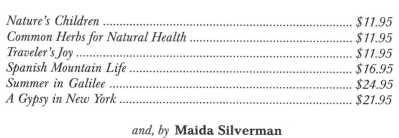